ADVANCE PR

QUARANTINE LIFE *from* (

"Lest we forget the lessons of our past, Kari Nixon reminds us—in poignant yet relevant detail—that we've been here before, and, more important, we can find our way out."

—Niki Kapsambelis, author of *The Inheritance: A Family on the Front Lines of the Battle Against Alzheimer's Disease*

"A brilliant look at the history of humanity through the lens of disease, this book is a must-read for anyone who has found depths of resilience and determination in this pandemic (and that's all of us). Smart, accessible, and downright funny, Nixon's *Quarantine Life* presents an in-depth archive of our collective past in order to better illuminate who we will be beyond just survivors of a pandemic. Her words make us reflect our own self-prioritization and adaptability, and, most important, have us believing we will come out of this better than when we entered."

—Aparna Shewakramani, TV personality

"I've interviewed over three hundred scientists for my show and read nothing but science books. Never have I met someone whose incredibly distinctive work became so serendipitously relevant and important at such a specific moment in time. Kari packed a wonderful overview of three hundred years' worth of literary accounts from humans impacted by various pathogens through modern history and mixed it perfectly with modern science to give us much-needed historical perspective on the present while providing balanced views on COVID and other current diseases and, perhaps even more important, a clearer outlook on the inevitable future. Whether you're into history, literature, or science, or just want to better understand the many frustrating and seemingly counterintuitive responses contemporary humans are having while experiencing their first pandemic . . . this is a book centuries in the making that is a must-read today."

—Shane Mauss, host of the podcast *Here We Are*

QUARANTINE LIFE

from

CHOLERA

to

COVID-19

WHAT PANDEMICS TEACH US ABOUT

PARENTING, WORK, LIFE, *and* COMMUNITIES

from the 1700S *to* TODAY

KARI NIXON, PhD

TILLER PRESS

New York   London   Toronto   Sydney   New Delhi

TILLER PRESS

An Imprint of Simon & Schuster, Inc.
1230 Avenue of the Americas
New York, NY 10020

First Tiller Press hardcover edition June 2021

TILLER PRESS and colophon are registered trademarks of Simon & Schuster, Inc.

For information about special discounts for bulk purchases,
please contact Simon & Schuster Special Sales at 1-866-506-1949
or business@simonandschuster.com.

The Simon & Schuster Speakers Bureau can bring authors to your
live event. For more information or to book an event, contact the
Simon & Schuster Speakers Bureau at 1-866-248-3049 or visit
our website at www.simonspeakers.com.

Interior design by Laura Levatino

Manufactured in the United States of America

1   3   5   7   9   10   8   6   4   2

Library of Congress Cataloging-in-Publication Data has been applied for.

ISBN 978-1-9821-7246-6
ISBN 978-1-9821-7247-3 (ebook)

For Flora and Zelda
Taller than the trees, bigger than the sky, and deeper than the ocean

———

And **because of** Mom, Dad, and Gracie
Because you loved me, I could love. Because you fought for me,
I found I could fight for others.

CONTENTS

CONTENTS

CONTENTS

ACKNOWLEDGMENTS

The Acknowledgment

No one has worked harder on this book (besides me) than my husband. In *Great Expectations* by Charles Dickens, the indomitable little Pip says to his love interest, Estella, "You have been in every line I ever read." It's cloyingly romantic. But perhaps the fact that you, Daniel, "have *read* every line I ever *wrote*," is even more romantic. This fact bespeaks labor, empathy, and a synergy of goals that is the love of real life, not of novels. This version of romance is an untiring, service-minded love that toils alongside, sometimes unglamorously. This love has seen you microwaving pizza while I wrote, or playing with the girls while I wrote, or buying groceries while I, you guessed it, wrote. It has seen you editing my grammar when my eyes were too strained from a day of researching. It has also fueled some of our amazing adventures, as you traveled with me while I studied old scientific documents and instruments in England, where you never once lamented the time spent so doing and, in fact, were joyfully eager to be such an integral part of my mind and thought. Perhaps most dear to my heart, this style of love has fueled our conversations for over a decade, as we chat about my projects and their trajectory over an evening cocktail, by a warm fire, surrounded by the much-too-many animals we've adopted. You listen, you think, and *we* dream of projects that I carry out but that we, together, envisioned and helped grow. Our talk never grows stale, because we travel the life of the mind hand in metaphorical hand, and there is always some unexplored nook or cranny that you brave with me. One day we'll grow old, but beside you, I'll always feel the child-like joy of discovery and investigation with a trusted, much braver friend.

Such is only possible *because you have read every line I've ever written*. Every. Single. One. You know what I know, and can theorize with me, remind me of evidence I've forgotten, and help me track down sources whose authors you remember sometimes better than I do. Your love is sometimes quiet, but it is always vast. It has shown me the depth of human goodness like a beacon.

Kven spør etter leidi når ein har slik vind![1]

Critical Acknowledgments

Just as I have so many friends and family who've shaped who I am and how I think about life, so too have a variety of scholars, some of whom I'm lucky enough to call my friends. In some cases, I will specifically name a scholar who has most heavily influenced my own learning on a given subject so that readers can dive more deeply into some of these historical figures and discoveries, should they choose. I refuse to pretend my thinking was created in a vacuum, for as I've already suggested—and as I will continue to insist—we are all connected. Beyond this, my desire for encouraging shared connection between seem-

---

1   Olav H. Hauge, "Du Var Vinden," in Olav H. Hauge, *Vakraste Dikt* (Oslo: Samlaget, 2014).

ingly separate communities extends to the Ivory Tower; there are some great scholars out there, doing great work, and this work shouldn't just be read by other academics. Whenever possible, I'll recommend some extra reading to you by scholars whom I find both incredibly bright and also accessible—scholars who want their work to influence the public, and whose work might just make the world a better place. But I'm only human, and it would be impossible for me to name every scholar who has influenced my thinking; there are scores of them, and I owe a debt of gratitude to each. Thank you also to my dissertation committee, whom I thank at great length in my academic book, but here I will simply say that I will always refer to you as the parents of my mind—the people who helped me gain a unique academic understanding about public society and the world that you personally know I so desperately needed in order to understand my private life. So thank you to Ross Murfin, Rajani Sudan, and Beth Newman.

Other Acknowledgments

Mike and Betty: You're my biggest cheerleaders. Mike, I think you're still the only nonacademic who has ever braved reading my dissertation! Both of you have always stood by me, encouraging me, setting up workstations for me, and asking about my work with more interest than almost anyone else. I guess that's where Daniel gets it. Thank you, too, for raising him so we could find each other.

To the now lifelong friends who have weathered highs and lows with me and stayed invested in friendship with me even when the necessary duties of motherhood pulled me off the radar for long stints, thank you for loving me and showing me a way outside my own critical self-perceptions. There is a saying in Norwegian: "Show me your friends, and I will show you who you are." Well, if there's any chance that you admire me as much as I admire you, then I can believe that

ACKNOWLEDGMENTS

I'm more than the worst I sometimes tell myself. So thank you, Jordan and Kathi Harp, Rupal Mathur, Amy Whitaker, Lorna and Chris Goldsmith & Co., Lori Stephens, Ben Jousan, Dustin Barth, Ashlee Hueston, Emily Merrell, Chelsea and Seth McKelvey, Anna Hinton, Meg and Charlie Wadle, Heather Flabiano, Mia Plunkett, Bonet Nuttall, Natalie Maddalla-Mulligan, Courtney Barajas, Elise Leal, Andy Christensen, Smokey Fermin, Allie Shook-Shoup, Bert and Jerusha Emerson, Casey and Liv Andrews, Jonathan and Stacey Moo, Tony and Amanda Clark, Beth Torgerson, Rob and Donna Fifield, Katie Larimer, Caitlin Tumlinson, and Brooke Kiener.

Thank you to Skogfjorden and Concordia Language Villages, for teaching me that we are all responsible for one another, even when I was an angsty teen and didn't want to hear it. You kept telling me, though, and soon it became as familiar as the beating of my own heart.

To my agent and friend, CeCe Lyra: There's a saying by the Persian poet Hafiz that reminds me of us: "Your heart and my heart are very old friends." It feels like I've always known you. Your spirit has been a blessing to my life, and I'm so grateful our souls found each other. Thank you for always being the cheerleader I probably need too much, and for being my friend *and* agent. And a huge thank-you for coaxing me to be open to a part of my writing life that I hadn't really dared to contemplate. Please, let's never forget about Nick. Or was it Nathan? Norman. It was probably Norman.

To Ronnie Alvarado: You and I are like cereal and milk, and your editorial mind is a perfect temper to my rambling hot mess of a mind that some might call creative. I never really felt like an "artist" until I caught myself frantically e-mailing you at all hours of the night, and I was so glad to know intuitively that you would always respond with patience and even-handedness. Sometimes I really felt, in those moments, that I must be hard to work with, but the gift you bestowed upon me was never, *ever* making me feel that way. Thanks for believing in this book!

INTRODUCTION

Death and taxes. There's an old saying that these are the only two certainties in life, that they're the only things we're guaranteed. To that list should be added "disease." Because to live a life without disease means having either perfect genetics or a perfect life somehow free from encounters with the disease-causing pathogens that are all around us. Such a superhuman has yet to exist.

There has never even been a time on this planet without bacteria and viruses—at least not while we humans have been around. For the entirety of recorded history, disease has loomed, a haunting shadow waiting to strike and decimate. Disease has *always* been a given, and the question of the next pandemic has never been "if." It has always been "when."

I am many things: a professor, a mother of two young children, an avid rescuer of far too many animals who are dubiously well-behaved. But more than anything, I'm a disease-lover. You heard that right: disease-lover. I mean this theoretically, of course. I hate being sick as much as the next person. Probably more, in fact. Although I'm a pretty basic white woman, I deeply believe it was I who first invented the "man cold." And yet if you met me on the street or in the store, before I tell you about my kids, my husband, or the books I've written, I'd be more likely to chat with you about my undying love of disease. Seriously—ask any of my family, friends, or students. I'm the disease girl. Because of some of my recent publications, I'm often jokingly referred to as the "syphilis professor" at my university, a title I accept reluctantly only because Group A streptococcus and tuberculosis are actually my favorite illnesses, *not* syphilis. I could fill a whole book with how I got here—how I became "the ~~syphilis~~ (*ahem*) streptococcus professor." There are lots of reasons I became the type of person I am, the type who wants to think about bodies when they're out of our control, when they're not behaving the way we'd like to think they "should." But that is a book for another day. For now, it makes more sense for me to explain not the how but the *why* of my disease fascination. This whole book, after all, is about how humanity's history of surviving plague after plague can help us, not just as society grapples with the COVID-19 pandemic but also for the next plague, and the one after that. Because remember, it's always a matter of *when*, not *if.*

The short answer about why I love disease: disease is people.

Here's the long answer: We care about disease only when it affects people (or sometimes when it affects the animals we love or rely on for sustenance). We can chart mortality statistics and map epidemiological spread. We can explain protein structures and methods of replication. We do all this, though, because a disease affects us and our loved ones. Even a plant virus will matter to us if it affects our food supply. But the random bacteria living on some algae in a nearby pond? Who cares? Until or unless it affects humans, that is. Perhaps you've never thought about it this way, but "disease" is literally simply a way of marking something happening to our bodies (or the bodies of plants or animals around us) that concerns or distresses us. With ever-advancing scientific and medical technology, it's easy to lose sight of this fact, or to assume that any given disease is some stable entity that exists out there, outside of us. You could say this is true of pathogens themselves—viruses and bacteria certainly do exist without us (although viruses must have *some sort* of host). But the *diseases* they cause—the things we name and treat as having some sort of independent existence—only in fact exist as defined against the idea of a sound human body that they invade and sicken. Thus, to name disease is to name ourselves, or at least some version of ourselves and our communities as we think they *ought* to exist (and no longer do). Cholera only exists as a concept because it destabilizes the idea we have of bodies *without* cholera—"well" bodies that define our norms. And quite often, this imagined "well" body or group is something we notice only when it's taken away from us through disease. Contagious disease is especially good at demonstrating this, because unlike cancers or heart disease, we can much more easily perceive that contagious illnesses come from external threats. Contagious disease in particular reveals the ways we have come to think of ourselves (I'm healthy, I'm active) and our communities (I'm connected with *this* group, not that one) as anything but stable factors of our identities. They are in fact fantasies, or desires at best, that disease—perhaps the most human thing aside from humans themselves—exposes as such. And when disease exposes these fantasies, we shiver in our vulnerability, certainly. But we're also motivated to adapt ourselves—to grow and change, and become a new, better version of who we've been. So for me, disease is only as horrifying as it is beautiful in its capacity to force us to reckon with who we really are, individually and collectively. In 2021, we stand at a historical advantage, too. If we confront this reckoning proactively, by learning from what previous generations of humans have had to face, our own reckoning might be a little less painful. We might just feel a little less naked and vulnerable when (not *if*) our time comes to face disease.

———

After the development of germ theory in the 1880s, modern Western medicine made huge inroads into the war against disease. Because of proactive warfare in the form of vaccines, and also through the creation of counterterrorism tools such as antibiotics, infectious disease has retreated from the front lines of public fears. In the last fifty years or so, it has been replaced by fears of the noncontagious: heart disease, diabetes, cancers, and dozens more. Contagious disease doesn't scare us today the way it did even seventy years ago, before the polio vaccine was invented. Ironically, our hard-earned confidence in the face of contagion has made us less prepared than ever to confront the "when" that we now face, which, at the time of writing this, is the COVID-19 crisis. After the pandemic itself ends, its repercussions will ripple outward—in the economy, in families, in product development, in supply chain management—for decades to come. Thus, even after COVID-19 is controlled, our medical privilege could very well be our downfall, because it is the very thing that has allowed us to forget what disease is like, and the damage that it does. And of course, there will always be another pandemic. Our assumption that we're magically impervious to disease has already allowed us to be caught unaware by the pandemic, as Westerners watched the disease's spread in Wuhan but generally didn't seem to believe it would be a threat in their communities. It also delayed many shutdowns and social-distancing efforts, as generational bravado about infection prevented us from really believing that we, too, could die from contagious illness. Yes, even in "the Land of the Free" hospital beds are finite resources, and doctors can be too sick to work.

So, we find ourselves oddly and suddenly (at least in our conscious awareness) connected to our ancestors who lived in terror during the 1347 bubonic plague, to the parents wondering whether to inoculate their children against smallpox in the 1700s, to the young adults who were mysteriously wiped out in the 1918 influenza outbreak. In 2020, we were stripped of the modern hubris that made us overly brave, and we now stand existentially naked and prone to the ravages of tiny, pathogenic particles.

But even now we have tools that bacteria and viruses don't have: emotional resilience, sheer grit, and single-minded determination. In the face of a deadly virus like Sars-CoV-2, the human body seems delicate—a just barely calibrated machine with its gears always on the brink of slipping, or worse, grinding to a halt. Humankind, however, has evolved to be the preeminent species on the planet not because of brute strength but because we're stubbornly determined to survive. To individual humans, the protein-spiked ball of the novel coronavirus is indeed formidable, capable of taking any one of us down, given the right circumstances. To the entire human race, however, the viral particles are specks of soulless computer code up against the tenacious spirit that domesticated everything from fire to farm animals. Delicate, frail, and vulnerable we humans may be, but we are damned stubborn, if nothing else. A quick note before we go on: I use COVID-19 intentionally throughout this book to refer to the *illness caused in humans and animals by* the pathogen, which I will refer to as either the novel coronavirus or Sars-CoV-2. Such a distinction also maintains medical and scientific accuracy.

Nationalism aside (and believe me, we'll get there—no book on global disease can sidestep the issue), the human race is one of relentless ingenuity and creativity. We are the species that decided jumping into the vastness of the ocean on so many pieces of wood seemed like a good idea (Hello, navies! Hey there, global trade!), who looked at a piece of grass and somehow determined it could be ground and cooked into something delicious (Oh hi, gluten-y goodness!), who needed to go faster and farther and so dug up trillion-year-old dinosaur juice and processed it into a completely different product that would change the world while simultaneously destroying it (Alas, fossil fuels!). As this last example indicates, we humans can be both our own greatest ally and our own worst enemy. No pathogen has succeeded in wiping us out yet, but COVID-19 is certainly giving us a run for our money. To be frank, I think we'll survive this, but the question we need to also be asking is, who will we be on the other side? Who do we want to be when we get there?

I believe that history holds the answer to these questions. Studying the past will show us not only how we can craft our biological survival as we weather the storm of the COVID-19 pandemic but also how to think ahead and become, if not the best, then at least a better version of ourselves as a whole—and not in spite of the novel coronavirus, but because of it. The novel coronavirus today—and hundreds of diseases from the past—can help us learn how to be and do better for the next plague, and the next, and the next.

The human race has managed to survive epidemic after epidemic, and while these crises left tragedy and trauma in their wake, they also made way for much-needed conversation, debate, and, in the best cases, widespread social reform. As much as we might see them as the enemy, microbial lives are intertwined with ours. Scientists even theorize that viruses developed from rogue pieces of human DNA that somehow gained independence—a sort of microscopic SkyNet event. Bacteria were likely some of the first living organisms to inhabit our planet at all. Of course, no one wants to die from disease, but there is a way to frame humanity's contest with microbes as a critical part of our strategy in paving a path forward, not just barriers to be bulldozed as we sally forth. In purely physical terms, it's now widely recognized that having "good" bacteria is essential to living a healthy life. In fact, scientists began to discover this in the 1890s, but scientific insight and broad public acceptance of an idea are often two separate happenings; only in the recent past have the two met, resulting in greater marketing of probiotics and other positive advances. We now recognize that we humans live interconnected lives with bacteria. Similarly, humans themselves developed *in tandem with*—not in spite of—viruses. As early as 2000, scientists discovered that critical bits of viruses were likely what allowed placentas to form, and the human race to progress. That is, viruses, these humble bits of code possibly derived from human DNA millennia ago, have, in some cases, worked their way back into the human genome, becoming a permanent part of ourselves once more. As one provocative *NOVA* article puts it, "Humans are, in a very real sense, part virus."[1] With that in mind, I would like to posit something radical here: that we see these pathogens as not just biologically intertwined with our individual and collective lives but as socially and emotionally intertwined with them as well.

Each time humanity survives an epidemic, we emerge on the other side of the crisis fundamentally different than we were before. Even in the present chaos of the coronavirus, we are all markedly more aware of the sheer number of things we touch, and the way touch unites us— for better or worse—to other humans. Gone is the mentality that we can exist as islands unto ourselves. The list of how humans have had to reassess our interactions is far-reaching. Parents have been forced to reconsider how highly they value daycare workers and teachers, communities have been asked to reconsider what is truly the "essential" work that society relies upon, and we've all been asked to stretch our needs for community and companionship to the utmost as we strive to ensure that such a community still exists. All this human change has come from a virus much, much tinier than a dust mite. If our privilege from Western medicine allowed the novel coronavirus to take us by surprise, the virus has nevertheless taught us a lot already. Priorities have been reevaluated, and huge numbers of people have been forced to examine the choices they've made on individual and community levels.

---

1   Carrie Arnold, "The Viruses That Made Us Human," *NOVA*, September 28, 2016, www.pbs.org/wgbh/nova/article/endogenous-retroviruses/.

By carefully studying the history of the people who've lived through plagues before us, we can avoid being taken by surprise again, while retaining the vital lessons pathogens can teach us. At the time of writing this, numerous studies on antibody creation after a bout of COVID-19 have left many disappointed—it appears that antibody numbers are not terribly robust some months after infection. And yet some scientists have hypothesized that T cells—which are essentially the long-term memory of the immune system—may be the key to COVID-19 immunity. I believe we need to be like T cells in terms of our social thinking: we need to invoke a long-term memory of human society. We need to dig deeply into the archives of human knowledge—knowledge from other eras when society didn't have pharmaceutical interventions for disease. These eras are going to more closely mirror what we'll go through when humanity encounters a disease it's never seen before, in the months or years it takes to develop treatments and vaccines.

The last fifty years of history are but a blip in human development, and one in which all our advancements have ironically given us knowledge of how to avoid pandemics but simultaneously robbed us of generational wisdom about what to do when they occur. We've decreased the threat of infectious disease in the developed world, that is, but in doing so have decreased our own ability to cope with rampant epidemics when they happen. The inverse is true, too. As little as a century ago, mortality rates from infectious disease were higher, but so, too, was familiarity with what disease really is and what it's caused by. People understood much more intimately what diseases looked like and what they did to the body. They also understood what it meant to exist—to simply *be*—while plague ravaged the world around them, with nothing to do but envision the world on the other side not just as a return to "normal" but as something better. Not only *can* we learn much, therefore, from the people who lived and died in these worlds but we *must*, or we have much more to lose than our lives. We risk losing the beautiful and vibrant elements that define humanity itself.

INTRODUCTION

I've said I'm a professor, and it's time to unpack this a bit more. I'm an English professor. Yes, take a moment. Spit out your drink in surprise, or whatever you need to do to take in this statement. Then come back to this paragraph, and I'll explain. Ready? Okay, then. I specialize in what's called the medical humanities, which can be described as a sort of "umbrella discipline" including medical ethics, the history of medicine and science, and medical representations in literature. For my part, I do a little of all of these. In fact, many English professors in the twenty-first century combine a healthy dose of philosophy, history, and literary studies to do their work. Most English professors also live by the adage "Everything is a text." In academic publications, professors routinely analyze newspaper articles and scientific treatises as much as novels and poetry. I have coauthored a book that, among other things, analyzes the language used on infant formula cans, and I've had students do projects analyzing the intake forms used in doctor's offices. "Everything is a text" also applies to our abstract world: our society, our norms, geographic boundaries, clothing, all of these things can be analyzed using the training English professors receive during their doctoral work (which generally includes historical, literary analysis, and philosophical training). So, while I have a PhD in literature and routinely teach in my literary specialty of the Victorian era, replete with all the Brontës and Austens and Eliots and Hardys you please, my research specialty from my graduate days was derived from exploring how authors like these responded to growing and changing scientific information about disease during their lifetimes. Thus, I'm equally as often teaching my medical humanities students to navigate and analyze WebMD pages as I am instructing them to use anthropological approaches to immerse themselves in the Victorians' medical world. These tools ask students to defamiliarize themselves with the assumptions we all make every day and to think like someone who has never lived in our world before. How would it look to them? What biases might they notice that we take for granted every day? In this book, I hope to impart some of these strategies to readers as well.

But first, it's important to state early and clearly: I will not be making health recommendations in this book. For one, I'm not, nor do I ever claim to be, a scientist. Yet I absolutely believe a literature professor like me has a lot to offer without needing to claim particular scientific credentials. What I see our world growing frustrated with (which I will address at length in the following chapters) is that even the world's best epidemiologists and virologists are dealing with something new, novel, and, at times, perplexing. None of us know perfectly what to expect, because we're in totally uncharted territory. The data about COVID-19 seems to change daily, and I see more and more people around me experiencing "data fatigue." I think, perhaps, more than data, we all want to know how to *feel*. And I think a long-term, T cell–like historical memory can help us calibrate our emotional response to COVID-19 as much, if not more, than scientific studies about the virus's epidemiological flow.

In the chapters that follow, I ask you to journey through time alongside me, getting to know the amazing personalities that contributed to our (perhaps overly) plague-free life as we know it, and who remarkably did so even as plague threatened to upend the world as *they* knew it. Along the way, I will offer tips—sometimes practical tips for physically and emotionally navigating these waters, sometimes philosophical or theoretical tips for making sense of the endless debates about ever-changing COVID-19 data and recommendations. As best I can, while never hiding my political leanings, I will attempt to make these tips nonpartisan, or at least to recognize the valid claims made by both sides in a partisan debate. Because I—like every other human on this planet—have my own political views and biases, I may not always be successful in my attempt, but I hope at least to demonstrate the sincerity of my efforts in providing insights into what we're living through—both the disease and the social turmoil—that can help any reader, not just those who already agree with me.

If I've learned one thing in my years of studying the social impacts of disease, it's that we live in a world where we're connected, for better or worse, to the people in our human community by the microbes that we share between us. And in times of contagious disease crisis, if we fail to recognize our shared connection, we are most certainly doomed, because our fates hang together, yoked by tiny particles that threaten us all. Scores of historical figures—both famous and obscure—have taught me as much. By learning the stories of those who lived before us, by educating ourselves about the worlds they inhabited and the viruses and bacteria that lived in, with, and through them, we can learn how to emerge from the novel coronavirus pandemic stronger than ever before and well prepared for the next new disease we will inevitably face. If we don't learn from their examples, however, I foresee a world adrift, damned by alienation from its own history, a victim of self-annihilation cued, rather than caused, by the novel coronavirus.

1

#LISTENTOWOMEN

Smallpox, Vaccines, and the World before Germs

1721

A walnut shell full of infected pus and women's intuition changed the world as we know it. In 1721, when Mary Wortley Montagu, an English ambassador's wife on a voyage to Turkey, saw Greek women saving their families from smallpox by having infected pus purposefully put into open wounds on their children's arms, she saw her chance to change the world—and she refused to let men ignore her. Her story, and several others like it, presents concise lessons that the history of vaccination can teach us in the time of COVID-19—messages that actually have nothing to do with vaccination itself, and everything to do with

Lesson 1: Looking for answers where you least expect them (aka Listen. To. Women.).

Lesson 2: Understanding that public health debates have always been about a tension between individual liberties and the collective good.

Lesson 3: Realizing that "choice" is a relative concept.

Montagu's story—and those of other women trying to protect their children from disease—is a helpful beginning point as we attempt to navigate plague survival, not only because she precedes other stories in this book chronologically but also for another important reason. Her experiences show us that before we can dive into the difficult work of survival and rebuilding, we first need to be sure that we're asking the right questions and looking for answers in the right places. The lessons derived from Montagu, in other words, help us calibrate our initial approaches to tough questions and even tougher conversations. But before we begin her story of courageous motherhood, I want to share another, more recent one that may seem unrelated but has helped me understand critical aspects of Montagu's own story from a very different vantage point.

Dublin
March 26, 1842

Ms. McCormick looked sleepily out the window, attempting to gauge, by the amount of light, what time it was. She squinted at the darkness; it was the middle of the night—maybe 2 a.m., if she had to hazard a guess. She could hear little Patrick wheezing in the bed next to her, and her heart hitched midbeat in her chest, hovering between instinctive parental panic—*Is he sick again?*—and seasoned maternal confidence—a little raspy breathing was nothing; he had just been treated in hospital for a suspicious cough, after all. He was probably still on the mend. Should she rouse him? She sat up, put her feet on the floor, and paused, wavering between these poles of certainty and fear while also weighing her divided physical loyalties—her own twelve months of sleep deprivation since Patrick's birth and her impulse to check on her baby.

Ultimately, the special cocktail of guilt and duty surging through her in the black darkness won out, and she lifted her baby from where he had been nestled. As her drowsiness melted away, she could now hear just how labored his breathing sounded. His back vibrated jerkily in her palms with every laborious drag of breath. What had begun as dutiful, better-safe-than-sorry wakefulness now crystallized into sheer panic as her eyes adjusted to the darkness and she could see him. As he strove to breathe, Patrick worked his tongue in and out of his mouth with a furious intensity that bespoke fever and delirium—that much was obvious even in a child this young. She'd never seen any baby do this—rolling the tongue up and down along the hard palate, in and out along the teeth, as if the organ were irritated. She'd never, in fact, until that moment considered the tongue to be an organ unto itself, and before she could fully piece together the raw ends of her alarm, she saw her baby boy as he was—a mere sack of organs, vulnerable to some horrible fever that was eating away at him before her very eyes. She put Patrick to her breast, relieved that he nursed readily. That had to be a good sign, she told herself, as she sent for the doctor and the apothecary.

The apothecary arrived first, but Ms. McCormick was glad to see anyone who could offer help. Although she was anxious for the doctor to show up, Mr. Brown was gentle, putting Patrick into a warm bath to soothe him, and administering emetics. When the doctor finally came, along with a colleague, Ms. McCormick was grateful to see them try everything medical science could recommend. She was a poor woman, and she hadn't been sure anyone would help her. The doctor disagreed with the emetics. Instead, he injected the baby with turpentine. By 11 a.m., Ms. McCormick was both comforted and despairing at the doctor's continued presence. She was grateful he was there, of course, tending to her poor baby, but the fact that he had remained so many hours meant this was serious. He wouldn't have stayed if he'd been woken at this time of morning for nothing. She looked out the window, hoping for a momentary distraction, watching the town go about its midday business while the atmosphere inside her walls was a nauseating mixture of monotony tinged with crisis; no one had moved, changed clothes, or taken a break for almost nine hours now, but everything had changed—everyone knew she might lose her baby. It was the secret no one whispered but everyone harbored. She glanced over her shoulder at the doctors. No one noticed her. How horrific to imagine that she, Patrick's own mother, was useless to him now! She who had given him life could only stand at the edges of the room wondering if he would die. The doctors were drawing blood from his arm while administering a mix of mercury and something else she couldn't recognize. Two hours later, there was still the sickening same-not-sameness as they bled her son's tiny body. (Bleeding was not much en vogue anymore, and perhaps it's for the best that Ms. McCormick likely didn't know that this probably meant the doctors were running out of ideas.) By evening, she had her boy back with her, nursing readily. *That has to be a good sign, right?* her inner voice repeated—this time, however, with a question mark added and an undertone of urgency, of desperation.

Dr. James Duncan, the man who eventually recorded this case, had arrived just after daybreak on March 26, and his case notes reveal the extent to which pre-twentieth-century society was collectively at the mercy of disease. Treatment after treatment was delivered to poor Patrick—everything as touchingly soothing as nursing with his mother and a warm bath to procedures that make the modern reader cringe (turpentine and mercury pumped into him, bleeding and laxatives draining his strength). These exhaustive efforts illustrate the very real desperation of doctors and families in this period to save their loved ones. Duncan's notes, published in his book *Illustrations of Infantile Pathology: Measles*, describe little Patrick McCormick as a "fine stout infant," and his nearly hourly journal of Patrick's progress, though largely optimistic in tone, ends abruptly with the baby's death during a series of violent seizures.[1]

Even 134 years later, one can visualize the "fine stout infant" readily. Duncan's copious notes make it inevitable that readers find themselves attached to the little boy, rooting for him and his mother, who, while standing across the bounds of two centuries from us, were nevertheless very real people who suffered greatly. While reading this for the first time, the mother in me stopped short when I came to the line announcing no further updates on little Patrick. I had assumed—as it seemed his own mother, the doctor, and the nurses also did—that he was making great progress. My heart caught in my throat when I read that he'd died after twenty-four hours' struggle with post-measles complications. I first read this mother's story while living in Washington State, an anti-vaccination stronghold, during a period when measles cases were on the rise. Her story reminded me of another mother who was born more than 160 years before her: Lady Mary Wortley Montagu. The two were separated by huge disparities in wealth and more than a century in time, but reading Ms. McCormick's experience allowed me to reflect on Montagu's in the shared light of their motherhood, and in the shared context of mothers' unique trauma in eras of high infant mortality. Though there were certain diseases associated with overcrowding that were less likely to affect the rich, in general, wealth made no great difference in terms of disease survival at a time when society had no real treatments for these ailments. What I'm about to tell you is the story of when Lady Montagu chose to do something very brave, but Ms. McCormick's story prompted me to ask: Did Mon-

---

1   James Duncan, "Illustrations of Infantile Pathology: No. II. Measles," from the *Dublin Journal of Medical Science*, 1842, housed at the Wellcome Library Digital Collections, https://wellcomelibrary.org/item/b21913110#?c=0&m=0&s=0&cv =2&z=0.0274%2C0.5779%2C0.8524%2C0.4313&r=0.

tagu really *choose* to, or did she *have* to, to protect her children? And if her different experiences as a mother affected her perspective about the options available to her, did it also impact where she sought answers?

London
April 1721

I envision Lady Montagu on her life-changing day in 1721, standing with the sort of feigned steadfastness that I can recall mustering when breastfeeding my daughters in public. I imagine her standing stiffly, with a kind of "fake it or you'll never make it and be taken seriously" hitch in her shoulders, mixed with a "come and fight me" set to her lip that I remember summoning up myself, in lieu of real bravery. The London air would have been just losing the last whisper of chilliness. Spring was steadily blooming as Lady Montagu stood alongside her daughter, waiting to begin. Among other witnesses there that day were four medical professionals. One, the surgeon Charles Maitland, would perform the procedure; the other doctors were brought from the College of Physicians as witnesses so that they could spread news of its success or failure. Lady Montagu was hardly the star of the hour—she was not at all what people had come to see—but my mother's heart zeroes in on her tension, her intense focus on trying to believe she was doing the right thing. Her pulse must have raced even as she kept that stiff upper lip—what if she was killing her daughter?

It was too late for fear now, however, as Charles Maitland approached three-year-old Mary (folks at this time weren't very creative in their naming practices) with a pus-laden lancet, made an incision on her arm, and spread the organic slime into it—slime that would have been harvested from an actively infected smallpox patient. No turning back now.

This day had been a long time in the making. Lady Montagu had recently returned from her travels abroad to Turkey (then known as the Ottoman Empire) with her husband, a British ambassador. While there, she observed that smallpox, a disease that intermittently devastated communities back home, seemed to be much less of a problem in these areas, places the British ironically viewed as "primitive" and "backward" (the British generally saw anyone who wasn't British in these terms, and they did even more so with regard to countries outside of Western Europe).[2] She inquired of local women in Turkey about this and was told about a strange process of preventive care, which she later witnessed. Her own experience with smallpox in 1715, which left her scarred, also likely made her keenly interested in investigating preventive measures. She explained the process she'd observed in Turkey in a letter home to her sister:

> *The small-pox, so fatal, and so general amongst us, is here entirely harmless by the invention of ingrafting, which is the term they give it. There is a set of old women who make it their business to perform the operation every autumn, in the month of September, when the great heat is abated.*
>
> *. . . The old woman comes with a nut-shell full of the matter of the best sort of small-pox, and asks what vein you please to have opened. She immediately rips open that you offer to her with a large needle (which gives you no more pain than a common scratch), and puts into the vein as much matter as can lye*

2　Diana Barnes notes this designation of "primitive" as well as "exotic." Diana Barnes, "The Public Life of a Woman of Wit and Quality: Lady Mary Wortley Montagu and the Vogue for Smallpox Inoculation," *Feminist Studies* 38 (2012): 330–62. Rajani Sudan elaborates on the latter particularly in her book *Fair Exotics: Xenophobic Subjects in English Literature, 1720–1850* (Philadelphia: University of Pennsylvania Press, 2002).

upon the head of her needle, and after that binds up the little wound with a hollow bit of shell.[3]

If you think the "vaccine wars" are intense now, characterized as they are primarily by groups of affluent white mothers who fear toxic chemicals, then buckle up. In her book *Alchemy and Empire: Abject Materials and the Technologies of Colonialism*, Rajani Sudan, a scholar of early modern British literature (and my mentor), explains that because Lady Montagu returned home from a nation the British saw to be beneath them, touting a foreign medical procedure—one traditionally presided over by women, no less!—she wasn't exactly met with open arms (or veins). But Lady Montagu persisted, inoculating her daughter in front of witnesses (the process wouldn't be called "vaccination" for some time) as proof that the procedure in fact happened, was no hoax, and, later, that it would protect little Mary from the dreaded smallpox.

There's an important point to make here before we go on, and it's one I learned from Sudan, whose *Alchemy of Empire* makes the following case in great detail. In many ways, Montagu's actions constituted colonization of medicine, or cultural appropriation, if you will. When Montagu brought the practice of "engrafting" or "inoculation" back to Britain, it was indeed met with a great deal of skepticism, largely because the procedure was developed in a foreign land. This Eastern process involved scooping matter from an infected smallpox wound, lancing the arm of a healthy patient, and smearing the matter in. It

---

3   Lady Mary Wortley Montagu, *The Turkish Embassy Letters*, Teresa Heffernan and Daniel O'Quinn, eds. (Ontario, Canada: Broadview, 2013), 125.

literally involved accepting a foreign element into one's body to protect oneself against fatal illness. In fact, Sudan describes Montagu as a woman whose self-avowed "patriotism" made her *willing* to "seek foreign techne in order to counteract smallpox."[4] Xenophobia (I told you we'd get back to this) had to be put aside if one wanted to live and, much more important, to save the nation as a whole from being overcome by disease. Montagu realized this. But these fears ran deep, as according to Sudan, "many Britons read inoculation as an unpatriotic act, a treasonous introjection of the elements of disease into what they perceived as the healthy corpus" of Britain.[5] It wouldn't be until the 1790s that the process would be more widely embraced, after Edward Jenner used the less virulent cowpox, derived from the wholesome dairy fields of England itself, to confer smallpox immunity.

So, while Montagu's openness ought to be applauded, it's also incredibly important to note the ways that this foreign, female technology was met with approval only when it was rebranded as a Western, male technology. Now, as many modern scholars take pains to point out, inoculation practices existed in many different cultures before Montagu's time—a 1700 letter from a British merchant mentions the practice as having existed in China for at least a century, and as early as 1731, employees of the East India Company noted its existence in India (though the practice itself was ancient). Cotton Mather mentioned learning about it from his African servant.

So, not only did inoculation-style techniques exist long before Montagu learned of them but she was hardly the first person to point it out to the British, either. Nevertheless, it was Montagu who refused to stop until doctors listened to her, and it was she who publicized and

---

4 Rajani Sudan, *The Alchemy of Empire: Abject Materials and the Technologies of Colonialism* (New York: Fordham University Press, 2016), 102.

5 Ibid., 121.

popularized the practice in Britain by virtue of sheer determination (and, let's be real, probably her aristocratic social position). To this day smallpox is one of the very few diseases considered to be truly eradicated from the planet, and even if it didn't quite start with Mary, her willingness to learn from other cultures played a large part.

And this is the lesson we can learn from Montagu:

LESSON 1:
Listen. To. Women.

Or, more to the point, we should always be looking for innovations from the people we might not be accustomed to listening to. As a medical humanist, I see my job as one that asks scientists and doctors to consider how they're framing questions, to see what implicit biases might be limiting their data analyses by limiting what they're even looking for in the first place. In this case, the bias seems simple, possibly preposterous: if a few men in the 1720s hadn't been willing to listen to a woman promoting foreign technologies, we might have been greatly delayed in widespread use of vaccines. However, this example seems straightforward only because we no longer blatantly ignore women's intelligence in the brazen way that was socially acceptable three hundred years ago. This doesn't mean that we are free of our own cultural biases.

One example of what this might look like in the age of COVID-19 is to consider that Western science often locates epidemic origins in non-Western spaces (Asia and Africa) and is quick to cite non-Western practices (eating certain meats, for instance) as their cause. It's not my place to judge the accuracy of these claims, but as a scholar of medical humanities, it *is* my job (and the job of many others who have made similar cases) to urge epidemiologists to check and recheck every layer of their quantitative research design—yes, even their statistical algorithms—for evidence of bias or oversight. As moral creatures, we have a responsibility to make absolutely certain that our repeated findings of Asian and African origins for diseases like Ebola, severe acute respiratory syndrome (SARS), Middle East respiratory syndrome (MERS), swine flu, avian flu, and COVID-19 are not a result of some social bias built into our statistics, because prejudice is possible even in math. The tools are only as good as the tools' users and their creators, and whenever your open-ended research turns up the same answer again and again and again, only the most reckless scientist or mathematician wouldn't cross-check their work to make sure this consistency is due to validated replicability (aka a "true" scientific finding) rather than to unintentional design bias misdirecting the results. To do this, however, requires assessing the roots of mathematics (the basis of epidemiology) itself, which runs counter to the ingrained adage that "math is universal." Careful "fact-checking" of our standards of epidemiological study design, then, might just involve looking to sources that we'd never expect—possibly even reconsidering how we've built the scientific method (which is another white, Western, male structure) to begin with. Does this mean I advocate an anti-scientific view of disease or that I aim to somehow debunk the findings of epidemiology? Not at all. But it does mean that some of the most groundbreaking medical discoveries of all time—those that foregrounded medical science as we know it today—came from listening to the most marginalized voices in the room, voices whose experiences were not mainstream and whose nontraditional insights may have very well saved the world.

―――――

Debates about inoculation began from the moment little Mary Montagu was publicly inoculated. The process was undeniably gruesome, and it was (understandably) hard to convince a society that believed in maintaining a strict balance in the body that opening up the body and smearing festering pus into it was somehow a safeguard against disease. The process took a somewhat better hold in the public mind when Edward Jenner further developed the inoculation process into what we now call vaccination. Etymologically, the term *vaccination* is derived from the Latin *vacca*, for cow, because Jenner theorized that using pus from the less dangerous but similar disease of cowpox might provide immunity to smallpox, but with fewer risks. The former technique of inoculation (which used smallpox pus) could in fact cause smallpox, which was of course often fatal. In a sort of medical colonialism, then, Jenner co-opted what was an Eastern, female-centric medical procedure, rebranded it as associated with wholesome English dairy farms, and then hailed the technique as the foundation of modern Western medical prowess.

Even once Jenner "invented" vaccination by branding it as English, however, many still resisted the idea of compulsory vaccination.[6] This was because compulsory vaccination was often mandated on quite young infants, who were exceptionally prone to the secondary infections they risked from incisions made with unclean lancets (antiseptic technology would be invented close to a century later). What's more, "public vaccinators" were obviously not marching into the homes of dukes and duchesses and snatching their babies for medical procedures against their will. The poor were much more susceptible to such infringements. As Nadja Durbach explains, "Who wielded the needle or lancet and whose body was marked governed how vaccination was experienced."[7] Among the wealthy, "cicatrix," or vaccination scars, became a sign of fashionable luxury—the rich could, after all, select their doctors, as well as the time of their vaccination. Everything was on their terms. For the poor, vaccination could quite rightly be seen as

6 Ibid., 110.

7 Nadja Durbach, *Bodily Matters: The Anti-Vaccination Movement in England, 1853–1907* (Durham, NC: Duke University Press, 2004), 5.

an infringement on their rights, as they were given no say about how, when, where, or by whom their children were vaccinated. Thus, from the very beginning, the vaccination debates took the shape of another lesson we'd do well to learn from:

LESSON 2:
Public health debates have always been about a tension between individual liberties and the collective good.

From as early as the 1850s, when England was first experimenting with compulsory vaccination, some families lamented that their bodily liberties would be sacrificed to the state by undergoing such an injection. Pro-vaccinators exclaimed that there were some cases in which public rights—such as the right not to be infected where said infection is avoidable by certain means—supersede individual liberties. Other sorts of private concessions to the public good, however, are easier to justify. Something like enforcing a noise violation involves asking someone to cease an unnecessary activity (playing loud music, for instance), whereas enforcing compulsory vaccination involves asking someone to undergo an activity that two parties disagree over the necessity of, and which one party may view as dangerous or harmful.

Although I've gone on the record as being pro-vaccination, it is not my intent to argue for or against vaccination here. To do so would easily fill its own book-length treatise. Rather, I hope to present the history of vaccination as a case study in how medical innovations arise when we're most effectively pairing science, creativity, and crowd-sourcing (**Lesson 1**). Secondly, as is the topic of this lesson, vaccination history can also show us when, where, and how the things we're debating are moot points, or givens that we need not spend further time arguing about. There are topics where the stakes are defined at the get-go, and in this case, we're wasting our efforts if we continue to debate the issue of individual rights versus common good. The definition of public health care during times of crisis, as the Hastings Center and others have affirmed, is simply the substitution of the common need—the benefit of the many—for the rights of the individual. You can argue that you *disagree* with public health's right to exist as a field because it replaces your individual rights with collective goals, but you *cannot* logically argue that public health during an epidemic *should* do something different—for doing so is the definition of public health crisis management. This is all it is, all it's ever done, and all it was ever intended to do. To avoid senseless debate about the wrong issues surrounding public health can save us time and energy that are best directed elsewhere, or at least allow us to hash out what we're really arguing about and embark on some sort of forward progress.

═══════

I haven't forgotten little Patrick. Lady Montagu's story was a necessary detour from the lesson Patrick's mother taught me as I read about her grief. To return:

LESSON 3:
"Choice" is a relative concept.

I've spent ten years of my life learning about disease in the nineteenth century, and a lot of my work has involved reading accounts—fictional and factual—about what it felt like to lose a loved one to infectious disease. But I'm also a mother of two young children, whom I love with a stereotypical cheesy fierceness. These accounts often come to us from male doctors rather than from bereaved mothers and wives themselves, but through the lines of the doctors' journalistic accounts I see the crazed grief of these women as vividly as if I were in the room with them. I've learned to read between the lines and understand the meanings behind seemingly insignificant notes: which details in a doctor's journal meant he was dealing with an impoverished mother; where that meant the baby slept (in the same bed with her, versus in a nursery, as would have been the case with a wealthier parent); which diseases themselves arose from living in overcrowded conditions; which were diseases of the wealthy; which interventions were given for the benefit of the mother's peace of mind; and which the doctor truly thought might help. The people who lived and died 160 years ago are as real to me as the people I see on the streets today, and I often furiously protect the reputations and perceived roles of authors and doctors I'm familiar with if I see them being misappropriated—they still have human dignity to me (this is going to come up in the longest footnote ever, in which I go down an investigative rabbit hole to find the source and motive of the uterus-pocket mystery in **Lesson 12**, a mystery involving a man I don't even really like), and I believe they'd want their memories preserved in certain ways, just as we do.

Of course, my ability to do this is often limited to relatively famous figures, about whom we know much. But when I read accounts like those of Patrick's mother, a poor woman living in a workhouse where only the most impoverished and desperate went, I'm struck by one resounding notion that rings over and over in my head with a ferocity: Patrick's mother wouldn't have believed a measles vaccine was a choice. I tell my students each semester that no one will ever be able to convince me that a mother who has watched her neighbor hold their baby while it died of polio would consider a vaccine a choice—they would consider it a necessity. Like so many other modern medical advancements, vaccines have partially given us the gift of forgetting: we've lost a generational memory of what it physically looks like to watch someone die of a bacterial or viral pathogen in front of our very eyes. This is not the slow hospice death of the modern world.

Death from infectious disease is messy. It is ugly. It is horrific. So while vaccine debates date back to the very introduction of inoculation to England, many of these early moments of vaccine hesitancy had to do with the risk of septicemia incurred by needles and lancets in an era before antiseptic technologies. That is to say that mothers who were not willing to vaccinate their children were often worried about secondary infectious diseases resulting from the vaccine process itself, and which were almost guaranteed death sentences if they occurred; I find this fundamentally different from many of the arguments made about vaccines today.

What the relativity of "choice" can teach us in the moment of this pandemic is that our belief that we have options about when, where, and how to socially distance is itself a conviction that might change in an instant if we were to watch somebody we loved die of COVID-19. That "choice" might not feel like much of a choice even in a different society, one that's more community-oriented than individualistic Western ones. It might not feel like a choice to essential workers, who must continue to do their jobs because they're required to do so by their employer, and because they may not be able to afford to decline or quit. The relativity of choice is nonpartisan. What seems like a choice to some may not actually be a choice for others. Recognizing this fact means asking everyone to examine the unquestioned assumptions that have led to their perspectives. To do so asks those who are hesitant to shelter in place to consider what might force their "choice" to become a "necessity." And it asks those who are pro-lockdown to be cautious in sharing memes criticizing those who aren't staying home. Such broad-stroke digital advocacy can have unintended consequences for those (usually marginalized and exploited labor forces) who don't in fact have the freedom of choice. Even though such memes are directed at those who actually *can* choose to lock down but refuse to do so, the message erases the perspective of a third group: those who *cannot* choose to stay home. These people may see such memes and feel at once scolded and also unseen and further marginalized by arm-chair public health advocacy that subtly denies their economically necessitated *lack* of choice. Humanities scholars Jenna Vinson and Clare Daniel put the matter neatly when they say that "the rhetoric of 'choice'" makes it appear as though we all have an "equal ability to make any given choice," while simultaneously "disguising" (here they quote two other scholars, footnoted below) "the ways that laws, poli-cies, and public officials differently punish and reward . . . different groups."[8] Choice itself is relative, then, and it is defined by privilege. In the next chapter, we'll explore some ways of breaking free of this myth and engineering a more equitable society of real choices for all.

---

8 Thanks to Jess Clements, my coauthor of another book, *Optimal Motherhood*, for this apt quote. Jenna Vinson and Clare Daniel, in part quoting Loretta Ross and Rickie Solinger, "'Power to Decide' Who Should Get Pregnant: A Feminist Rhetorical Analysis of Neoliberal Visions of Reproductive Justice," *Present Tense* 8 (2020), www.presenttensejournal.org/volume-8/power-to-decide-who-should-get -pregnant-a-feminist-rhetorical-analysis-of-neoliberal-visions-of-reproductive -justice/.

2

RISKY BUSINESS

The Question of Keeping Nations Thriving While People Die

―――

1722

Step 1: Install a sash window that opens upward (rather than the outdated casement windows, which open outward).

Step 2: Hang a basket on a rope. Lower rope out of window for grocery delivery. *Et voilà*: Contagion avoided, food procured.

Let's get right to it. Especially in the aftermath of the novel coronavirus, what we all really want to know is: What can we do to avoid getting sick? Surprisingly enough, one of the earliest novels in English—written by a humble son of a tradesman, no less—provides us with pretty useful answers. The example above comes from the work of Daniel Defoe, who with this description all but invented contactless food delivery. Aside from being a successful merchant, Defoe wrote tirelessly, endlessly. He wrote whatever anyone would read or pay him to write; think Alexander Hamilton in the musical *Hamilton*. In addition to his work writing pamphlets and other nonfiction, he wrote many novels, including *Robinson Crusoe*. When a smallpox plague ravaged London in 1721, Defoe did what he did best: he immediately wrote two books about plague, probably to reflect on and share information about the local recent experience with disease. Using both a fiction work, *A Journal of the Plague Year*, and a nonfiction manual (which contains a fictional play—go figure), *Due Preparations for the Plague*, Defoe explored what epidemics do to communities and gave his readers tips for surviving, focusing specifically on how to keep economies thriving while maintaining social distancing.[1]

It's hard for many of us to imagine now, but the novel as a type of literature didn't always exist. Scholars argue endlessly about exactly which novel was the very first one in English, but most people generally agree that the media form emerged in Britain and America around 1720, and few could deny that Daniel Defoe, son of a tallow chandler, was at least one of the English language's first novelists.

Yet although *A Journal of the Plague Year* is technically a novel, it doesn't read much like ones we'd recognize today. In fact, Defoe's "novel" is fairly identical to the nonfiction technical manual *Due Preparations for the Plague*, and both were published at about the same time. In *A Journal*, a narrator named H.F. (who is a merchant like Defoe) wanders the city of London and struggles to keep both his business and his body alive while he watches the daily decimation of

---

1 Versions of my interpretations of Defoe's plague writings have also appeared in both scholarly articles and in my 2020 book: Kari Nixon, "Keep Bleeding: Hemorrhagic Sores, Trade, and the Necessity of Leaky Boundaries in Defoe's *Journal of the Plague Year*," *Journal for Early Modern Cultural Studies* 14 (2014): 62–81; Kari Nixon, *Kept from All Contagion: Germ Theory, Disease, and the Dilemma of Human Contact in Late Nineteenth-Century Literature* (Albany: SUNY University Press, 2020).

the city and its populace around him. *Due Preparations* takes the narrativized "survival tips" featured in *A Journal* and presents them as more of a straightforward guidebook, with less plot structure, except for a prolonged closet drama at the end of the work in which a family considers how to prepare their souls for the afterlife. But both works more closely resemble a slew of mortality statistics with a smattering of instructive guidelines for survival rather than any kind of story with a plot. In *A Journal of the Plague Year*, there is admittedly a narrator who wanders about the city making observations, but he functions mostly as a vehicle for communicating the same mortality statistics and guidelines that Defoe presents in his own voice in *Due Preparations*. What could be so important that Defoe wrote two books with practically identical messages, you ask? The main things he harps on repeatedly in *A Journal* are:

Lesson 4: **Quarantine doesn't work—at least not like you think it does; instead, social distancing is our best weapon.**

Lesson 5: **Like it or not, we need economies.**

Lesson 6: **Statistics are our frenemies, so no, risk elimination isn't actually possible.**

More than perhaps any other historical figure covered in the present book, Daniel Defoe provides us with concrete, practical tips for surviving the plague physically—and still having a functional society on the other side of the crisis. As such, this chapter will be the closest I come in this book to stating anything even remotely like a public health recommendation. Even so, these moments are still intended more for the purposes of how to understand or live with these recommendations than to weigh in on any science. For, aside from mortality numbers, Defoe himself didn't have anything like the epidemiological science we know today. He simply had what he saw in front of him, day in and day out, just like you and me. I'll go even further and say that this is even the experience of the skilled epidemiologist or mathematician, who perhaps has access to, and a better understanding of, data than you or I but who nevertheless, in 2020, arrives home at the end of another lonely day of social distancing to a child or children whose worlds have been turned upside down. Even for such experts, mathematics is not a sufficient answer in the face of a child's emotional turmoil. Defoe's lessons knit together the practical and the existential in ways uniquely poised to help fill this gap.

The servant girl at the Pied Bull Inn shook herself out of her daydream with a start—she had completely forgotten about their latest guest.

The question was repeated in her direction: "Where is he?" She tried to think of the last time she'd seen him as she absentmindedly wiped some crumbs off a table. A man had arrived late last night, looking like someone who was trying to exude too much confidence as a disguise for simmering panic. She had peered over the innkeeper's shoulder to catch a glimpse at the traveler—no one ever liked nervous-looking travelers, but especially not these days with the plague going around. The staff at inns that were still operating had to guess as well as they could about who was well and who was ill. Most of the time, it felt like the best anyone could do was stare hard into the eyes of the would-be guests and silently ask, *Are you hiding something?*

By the time this particular guest had arrived, the inn was nearly full. "We've only got the attic," she'd heard the innkeeper grumble, and then, of course, it had been her job to lead the newcomer up to the dank room with a candle. She recalled that he didn't look like the type of fellow who would be used to sleeping in attics, and as they made their way up the stairs, he seemed reluctantly resigned to the bleak lodgings rather than grateful for a roof over his head—a sure sign he was something of a gentleman, she had thought to herself.

"Well?" She looked up, realizing that she still hadn't answered the innkeeper about the man who had arrived last night. He wanted to know where he was. She fumbled with an empty ale tankard near her and it dawned on her. *Oh no . . .* The poor fellow had sent her to bring him a glass of ale. She had gotten distracted by her other duties downstairs and had forgotten. In fact, she realized that she hadn't seen him since she'd led him to the room. It was well after morning, and he should have risen by now. The innkeeper had already leapt up the stairs by now, and she hurried after him, arriving in time to share in his horror. The man was no longer a man but a corpse. Her stomach churned: plague had arrived in their humble inn, and she had personally led it up the stairs.[2]

The narrator, H.F., recounts this instance in *A Journal* (he notes that the maid and many others in the inn died quickly afterward), because for Defoe, it is obvious that

LESSON 4:
Quarantine doesn't work—at least not like you think it does; instead, social distancing is our best weapon.

According to H.F. (and Defoe, in his own voice in *Due Preparations*), forcing people into quarantine is a fool's errand. In the world of *A Journal*, the narrator explains that town magistrates would enforce the "shutting up" of houses that had plague victims. These houses would

---

2   All narrative elements are adaptations of incidents found in Daniel Defoe, *A Journal of the Plague Year* (Oxford, UK: Oxford's World's Classics, 1990). This moment is found on pages 71–72 of this edition.

then be monitored by "watchmen" to see that no one went in or out. But over and over (and over and over!), H.F. recounts that when a house was forcibly shut up, the inhabitants would simply rebel and "break out" (his words), usually in a hysterical state from having been jailed in their own home. In their frenzied escape, Defoe argues that these people spread the plague more rapidly than ever. Defoe repeats these instances so many times that they become a bit ridiculous. Whenever I read the book, I can't help but imagine cartoonish figures running in circles, flailing noodle-arms, mouths frozen in an "O" of panic. I think this hint of the ridiculous was quite intentional on Defoe's part. Defoe was after all an accomplished novelist. So I have to believe that if he went to the trouble of penning this sort of incident over and over again, at a time when writing practices were much more laborious than they are today (quill pens and whatnot), he had a clear motive for doing so. And I think the reason is this: Defoe wanted to drill it firmly into his readers' heads—through mind-numbing, almost ridiculous repetition if by no other means—that Quarantines. Don't. Work. Period.

Before you throw down this book in disgust (or triumph, depending on your opinion about the COVID quarantines you've no doubt lived through), pause for a second, because there's more to say, and the matter is a bit more nuanced than you might be thinking. Defoe doesn't exactly say that quarantines are useless; instead, he emphasizes that self-quarantine is the only viable method for disease control. Defoe implies that there must be individual buy-in and consent to quarantine for it to be effective. H.F.'s insistence that the forcible "shutting up" of houses results only in frenzied flight makes this point clear enough. Throughout *A Journal*, Defoe repeatedly portrays the impossibility of fully enforcing mandated quarantine, with H.F. explaining to the reader that there was simply no end of things a family or individual would do to get out. Frankly, when under mandatory quarantine, a family had nothing but time to plan their escape. H.F. recounts stories of more than one quarantine guard being murdered or threatened with murder in the book. "Quarantine guard" is starting to sound like a heck of a gig, eh? But in all seriousness, Defoe uses such instances to point out the sheer difficulty of even recruiting enough quarantine guards to accept such a hazardous job, money aside.

Defoe is ever the pragmatist and makes the point that, like it or not, people must consent to how they're treated, or they *will* find ways to resist. In fact, Defoe suggests that such resistance makes disease spread harder to contain than if nothing were done at all: some previously quarantined people try to go underground, exposing others as they pretend not to be infected, while others simply panic and run, throwing caution to the wind as they go into full-on fight-or-flight mode. Defoe explains that mandatory quarantine did nothing "at all" except to "make the people desperate, and drive them to such extremities as that they would break out at all adventures . . . [and] those that did thus break out spread the infection farther by their wandering about."[3]

———

George felt his jaw tighten as he watched the man slowly track the red paint up and down and then sideways on his front door, in the mark of a cross. They'd asked him not to watch—the alderman and the watchman, that is—since it made the poor painter boy nervous, and it wasn't his fault he had to earn his bread by marking quarantined houses. But George hadn't budged.

"If you're going to make me a prisoner in my own home, I'll at least look i' the eye o' those that woul' be mae jailers," he had growled.[4]

Fanny, the maid, had fallen ill three nights ago, and in spite of all George's efforts to hush the matter up, he and his family had been ordered to quarantine.

———

3 Defoe, *Journal of the Plague Year*, 53.

4 This is adapted from a scene in ibid., 122–23.

"The death o' us, tha'll be," he had roared, "to be shu' up wi' the plague. We's that well ought to be let out, else she ought to leave us." No one had dignified him with a response. These were the rules. And so the paint boy had come, and now he backed inside the threshold as the door was closed and a padlock was placed on it. But George had a plan.

"You'll ha' to fetch her a nurse," George hissed at the watchman through the window.

"George, you been already told that there'll be no nurse brought into a den of plague."

"I'll let her die up there." His eyes flashed defiantly at the watchman.

"She's like to die no ma'"—the watchman began, but George's words stormed past his own, trampling them as though they'd never been uttered.

"She's four stories up—in the garret—and we'll none o' us go near to her. I'll no' go, nor will we bring victuals to her door. Bring a nurse or consent to her death," he growled.

"I—" But the watchman gave up. Everyone knew it was no use arguing with George, and while he knew the girl's death wouldn't really be his fault, still the thought of her starving to death alone, with no one to even hear her cries, was too much for him. One nurse couldn't do much harm in spreading the plague, could it? Not if she was shut up with the girl, he reckoned as he trudged down the muddy street to fetch one.

George lost no time. He had but a few minutes while the watchman was away to break down part of the wall that separated his home from his storefront. No one had thought to lock the shop doors. He and his family escaped their prison the next day, leaving, as H.F. recounts, "the nurse and the watchman to bury the poor [girl]; that is, throw her into the [dead] cart."[5]

---

5   Ibid., 52.

In fact, H.F. likens mandatory quarantine to "prisons without bars and bolts," meaning that it achieves precisely nothing in the realm of containment.[6] In short, people must consent to what is being done to their bodies. Of course, there is always that necessary tension between the collective health and individual rights that is an unavoidable tenet of public health (**Lesson 2**). But we need not try to apply his argument about quarantine consent to something like debates about mandatory vaccinations. This is the beautiful simplicity of Defoe: that he makes no moral judgment in his works, only pragmatic claims.

———

Well, Defoe may not criticize, but I will. I think that those of us (and I'm one) who have become fixated on the idea of consent in the last few years (How long does it last? Must it be reinstated with changing circumstances? How often? Can it be revoked?) must be willing to at least see the relevance of the sort of consent we've been discussing in the post #MeToo era—that is, sexual—to other issues of control over bodies. I think that, ethically, Defoe has a real point. Even while I recognize that public health ethics are ultimately about a public good over personal liberties, I do think, at least for argument's sake, we have to be willing to admit that there are some decently good—or at the very least, deeply human—reasons that people do not react well to the idea of forced quarantines.

So if we pretend that we cannot even see the rationale for these reactions, we aren't discussing the issue in good faith. We may believe that public good supersedes individual liberties in the case of mandated quarantine, but I believe in that case we must simultaneously acknowledge that mandatory quarantine produces the very resistant reactions Defoe predicted, and with some decent consent-based reasoning. And

---

6   Ibid., 53.

if we acknowledge this point—and I think it's pretty irrefutable—then we should not react with disgust to those who are opposed to quarantine. Frankly, I think that liberals (and in case it isn't obvious by now, I'm a liberal) should give some credit to those on the right who by and large may have grumbled about shelter-in-place mandates in America but ultimately often conceded and played by the rules of public health. Absolutely, there are many exceptions to this generalization, but the most memorable examples of this sort of blatant, loud resistance circulated on YouTube and Twitter were exactly that—the loudest protestors. Therefore, there almost certainly is a much quieter majority of people who disagreed with and disliked the idea of mandatory quarantine but generally played by the rules. In the case of America, however, this was too little, too late. Delayed quarantines contributed to the false notion, usually on the right, that such efforts didn't "work." For both sides, then, I urge giving the benefit of the doubt, both to individuals' compliance struggles and also to collective recommendations for public health. A little more trust—on both sides of the aisle—might go a long way toward helping another lockdown (whenever it might next be needed in human history) happen more quickly, and to be met with more appreciation and recognition of the real impact of quarantine on families. The two factors, I think, would facilitate each other. If people felt their efforts would be appreciated, they might be more willing to commit earlier on, and vice versa.

You'll hear me say this a lot in the coming pages—almost as frequently as Defoe depicts his runaway quarantine patients—but I have been disturbed more than anything in 2020 by the polarization of American society, and throughout this book I will be urging all readers to meet in the middle and see the value in portions of the opposing side's perspective. Perhaps this will make me unpopular with both groups, but it's an important enough ethical task to me that I'm willing to take that risk and be vulnerable in the name of asking you (all of you) to re-recognize our common humanity.

It should also be recognized, though, that our so-called mandatory quarantines in America were rather loosely enforced—no one was physically boarding up our houses and guarding them, as Defoe describes in *A Journal*, making the quarantine "mandate" more of an honor system—which, by definition, requires consent to opt into at all. We've come full circle, then, and technically, we've done this part of quarantine correctly in 2020: we may not have gotten user buy-in emotionally, but our "honor system" quarantine did require consent, even if it was grudgingly given. For Defoe, this is about as good as you can get with quarantine. More buy-in might have been desirable, but going about that is a health communication issue, to be covered in a later chapter.

————

Martha's hand shook a little as she marched down the street to purchase a roast for the Sunday meal. She was scared to be around people in the marketplace.[7] As she waited her turn, however, she was reassured by the butcher's procedures. She watched him carefully hang up the joint of meat on a hook, and she watched the customers then take their orders from the hook, not from his hands, to avoid contact. She also noticed the customers' coins were placed in a vat of cleansing vinegar instead of into the butcher's hands themselves. He then only took the money out at a later time, when one could at least hope it was cleansed of disease. She craned her neck, trying to see more while still maintaining her distance. She could tell by the interactions as well that the butcher was requiring his customers to use exact change, so that there was no exchanging of money required in the moment of purchase.

Defoe sprinkles his story with compelling moments like these,

---

7 Ibid., 78.

which are nearly identical to signs in stores during 2020 asking for exact change, and curbside pickup of goods. While we obviously got around to implementing these risk mitigation tactics, how much faster could we have been if there had been more awareness that this was codified for us in a book written three hundred years ago for just this moment?

One reason I find studying past epidemics to be of such importance to our present moment is that for the vast majority of human history, people didn't have pharmaceutical interventions to use against disease. There were only behavioral means of controlling disease spread. Because we've been lucky enough to live in an era of antibiotics and modern medicine, we've largely forgotten that we *can* use nonpharmaceutical interventions to control epidemic spread. Because behavioral changes were some of the only tools available in 1722, Defoe is keen to focus on describing what he believes will be useful, and aside from consenting to quarantine, he emphasizes social distancing.

For Defoe, first giving families themselves a chance to deal with infection by a means of their choosing—possibly by sending the sick person to a "pest house" (in our world, this might look like a special wing of a hospital) instead of mandating a forcible quarantine—might keep families from resisting and hiding infection within their homes. This could then reduce the overall infection rate of families "shut up" together and thereby infecting one another. So, the first thing of import for Defoe is to get a relative sort of buy-in to a personal decision to quarantine, whether at home or in a hospital.

But beyond simple self-quarantine, Defoe does a great job of envisioning what necessary day-to-day interactions could look like as safely socially distanced activities during plague, with anecdotes like the one that started this section. Recall his beta version of contactless delivery at the opening of this chapter. In 2020, it took a while for society to realize we could use grocery and food delivery more broadly to mitigate contact with one another, and to realize we could do all this via contactless methods. Perhaps if we had been a bit more attuned to the lessons from the past, we'd have been a little quicker about implementing these adaptations. As we all know by now, a few days' delay can cost us. Similarly, this would have made quarantine more bearable earlier on, and perhaps increased its adoption.

Of course, there are real and important class concerns associated with opting into delivery methods—the delivery personnel and those who stock and package our products must, after all, work to provide those who can afford it with this sort of contact mitigation. Even in 1722, Defoe was aware of such class-based ethical issues. In *Due Preparations*, he creates a thirteen-point list of how he envisions handling the poor and marginalized—especially and including convicts and children—to better protect the safety and social distancing of all. Defoe wisely points out that caring for the poor, for children and particularly orphans, and for those who are jailed is actually a critical part of saving all of us from plague.

Of course, there are many socioeconomic, regional, and supply chain factors at work here, but, as Defoe so deftly states, "if the poor could live within doors, as the rich may, the poor would be as safe as the rich are, but that necessity that sends them abroad to get their bread brings them home infected."[8] Translation: not being able to afford contactless grocery delivery and/or not being able to avoid going to work (which is how people can afford groceries in the first place) is one reason why lower socioeconomic groups are more prone to epidemics.

So how do we engineer a fix for this? Well, where there's a will there's a way. I don't claim to be a business guru or an economist, so I won't claim to know exactly how we might go about rendering universal contactless purchasing as an accessible service for all. Instead,

---

8   Daniel Defoe, *Due Preparations for the Plague, as Well for Soul as Body* (London: J. M. Dent & Co., 1895), 80.

I will quote Andrew Yang, former presidential candidate and proponent of universal basic income, to support my point that it's possible to bring this about if we as a society make it a priority. In his 2020 campaign, Yang's support for universal basic income for all citizens, provided by the government, was met with skepticism. During the 2020 COVID-19 shutdowns, however, stimulus checks were sent out to nearly all qualifying US citizens, at which point Yang noted, "What seems [now] to be marginal or overambitious is going to become common sense pretty quickly."[9] Yang's entire platform in the 2020 election cycle was that capitalism can be reimagined to better serve humanitarian interests. There's of course room for debate on this point, but his method of reenvisioning things we assume are a "take it or leave it" matter is the kind of thinking that's going to see us through pandemics with our society—and our humane instincts—intact. Speaking of economic stimulus, perhaps more than even his insistence on quarantine methods, Defoe's most repetitive point in both *A Journal* and *Due Preparations* is that

LESSON 5:
Like it or not, we need economies (Don't @ me).

Thomas rubbed his bad leg as he thought. It was a habit of his when he was worried, planning. Like his brother John, Thomas had been a sailor. At least, he had been until he hurt his leg. He relished the bracing clip of the salt air, though, and had stayed at least adjacent to the profession, becoming a sailmaker. John had been injured, too, but had only enough training to become an assistant baker. Sometimes

9   Ishaan Tharoor, "The Pandemic Strengthens the Case for Universal Basic Income," *Washington Post*, April 9, 2020, www.washingtonpost.com/world/2020/04/09/pandemic-strengthens-case-universal-basic-income/.

Thomas wondered if John missed being on the docks—at least there one could imagine freedom, even if they couldn't afford to go anywhere or do anything in particular besides try to survive.

"I'll be turned out of my lodgings, I will, John, if the plague comes to this neighborhood." John was silent. The light, scraping sound of Thomas's rough hands running back and forth over his pant leg was the only sound in the room. Thomas glanced at Richard, sitting behind John. Richard was by far the most serious and taciturn of the three—he was unlikely to weigh in. Thomas dropped his hand and resolved to break the silence himself. They had to have a plan.

"They say I go abroad every day to my work, and it will be dangerous; and they talk of locking themselves up, and letting no Body come near them."[10] Richard grumbled, while John shifted uneasily in his chair. What could any of them do? It was easy for the rich to flee to the country, but they had hardly anything saved and had to keep working to pay rent. And yet here were the landlords, shunning them for earning their keep.

The brothers eventually packed up and left for the country. On a large scale, such flight *from* cities, as Defoe points out, only puts the health of more people at risk. Enabling the ability of *everyone* to shelter in place is a critical means of ensuring compliance with protocol that can contain infection.

———

Defoe was insistent that economies are a necessary part of human society, even during (perhaps particularly during) times of plague. Of course, Defoe was a merchant, so his bias is showing here. But Defoe demonstrates a surprising ability to balance his entrepreneurial interests with his belief in a moral obligation to promote economic support

---

10 Defoe, *Journal of the Plague Year*, 122. This dialogue is a direct quote.

systems for those in need of them. And, ultimately, I think Defoe has an important point to offer us in this regard.

To support his ideas about economies, Defoe uses a metaphor of *open flow*, a concept that was very common during his time. Some readers might be familiar with the medical notion of "humors" from the early modern and ancient world. These were believed to be four different elements inherent to every human body. The balance of these elements was critical, as was their ability to flow freely. Stagnation of any one element was considered dangerous. In *A Journal of the Plague Year* specifically, Defoe applies this notion of fluidity to his arguments about the economy (one could argue he applies it to all elements of plague responses, in fact). For Defoe, the economic element of society must have even, ordered—and continuous—flow so that human bodies can also continue to "flow" (by which he means survive at all, by having food to eat, shelter to protect them from the elements, etc.). In a way, Defoe reconfigures the individual bodily humors from the medical world as a miniature model for how the world at large should work. In this larger world model, he presents human bodies collectively as one humoral element and the economy as another. He posits that the two must be balanced in power, and they must flow freely, independently, and concordantly with one another. This would mean, for instance, we ought not to stop up the economy entirely or shut up human bodies in mandatory quarantine. Defoe's notion of balanced flow would look something like Andrew Yang's idea of "human-centered capitalism" in our day and age. For Defoe, economies and people are equally important, and neither can exist without the other. Economies are necessary because they serve the people who sustain them with their bodies.

For some readers, this conclusion seems obvious. For some others of us, however, I would venture to say that capitalism and corporate enterprises run amok in the developed world have made it all too easy to want to throw the proverbial baby out with the bathwater.

Peak capitalism and all its evils have made it far too easy to assume we don't need economies at all. Because free market capitalism has been given far too few restrictions, particularly in America, many of us wish we could eschew the system entirely—myself included, at times. But taking a step back, it's very likely that we would problematically and unthinkingly doom the overall flow of goods and services if we scrap capitalism entirely. The market economy is a fundamental requirement of society, because it is the only way by which citizens can exchange their personal property (this includes their time and skills) for other things that they need for continued survival. It does seem to me that these exchanges are what make up a society to begin with and make its flow possible.

Under capitalist models, the individual is able to exchange their goods, labor, or time for other things. Most people probably prefer this freedom of choice, even if they can recognize that capitalism needs more checks and balances. If you're still unconvinced, that's fine, but I would at least urge you to see that since Western society has set up the system of free enterprise that we have so far, you might more readily understand why a single mother working a job in the service industry opts to go to work instead of self-quarantining—her kids survive on those tips. And we all survive on groceries, so someone needs to work the jobs that cultivate those, or society will actually fall apart. I don't know about you, but I don't know how to forage in the wilderness for food. So even if you remain committed to the ultimate long-term goal of dismantling capitalism, we all still have an immediate obligation to those who are absolutely dependent on its continuation in the present moment. They are the same people whom we unthinkingly depend on for our own subsistence, and so those people ought to be compensated, and more fairly than they often are. To have savings to live on is a luxury only a few in the middle and upper classes can afford. Most people rely on their hourly or tip-based wages, and frankly, most of us rely on that lesser-compensated work in the supply chain. So, at least for the time of this writing, I find Defoe's point to be absolutely spot-on. The economy must flow, and we should find ways to allow it to do so using fair compensation models and safe workflow chains.

Does that mean economies are more important than people, as some politicians have suggested? Not at all. Recall that a keyword in the metaphor Defoe relies upon is "balance" of humoral flow; economies and people are intertwined. Make no mistake: I'm a proponent of democratic socialism as seen in countries like Norway, where the quality of life is very high—but both proponents and opponents of socialism often neglect to mention the fact that Norway is a capitalist country as well. Sure, health care and education are subsidized heavily by the government—they're even free in many cases—but huge corporations like Statoil still make billions of dollars in Norway, much as Berkshire Hathaway profits in Nebraska. Now, Norway is no utopia, but their high quality of life, in my opinion, has been attained not through self-satisfied stagnation (to call back to Defoe) but because of the consistent and constant debates about how best to keep things improving—or flowing—toward a better future. There absolutely is a capitalist means that can make contactless delivery accessible for all, just as there are means toward better compensation of the employees that are truly essential to our collective survival. Among the many other goals of this book, one major object of mine is to inspire readers to think about what that might look like and how it might be implemented. If Defoe's insistence on balanced flow demonstrates anything, it's that keeping society flowing (if you're not sick of that word yet) is a communal job, and we all have something to offer. There are absolutely important roles for everyone—scientists, professors, business owners, economists, mechanics (remember the window pulley from *A Journal*?), artists, and countless other professions—to play in reimagining our world as healthier and safer for us all.

The story of the three brothers from *A Journal of the Plague Year* makes it clear that economic and class differences greatly determine our *ability* to respond to epidemics. Of course, issues like access to groceries and widespread health care are items we should have already been reimagining. But COVID-19 has become the inevitable rallying cry of a sick society, and we all have a role to play in healing it and bettering it for the future. It's time to get rid of the "handing it off to the experts" mentality. We all have something we can contribute. Scientists can invent vaccines, but they aren't equipped to figure out why this city or that state handled its distribution improperly. Doctors can sometimes use ventilators to help save the lives of those suffering from COVID-19, but they may not have any clue why their region doesn't have enough ventilators to begin with. More than anything, when I read about scientific innovations—particularly in medicine—I'm struck by the sheer creativity required to simply consider new paths and avoid the well-worn ones. Take for example, phage therapy, which involves reprogramming a virus to kill bad bacteria. Somebody somewhere had to think way outside of the preexisting box to come up with that one. That novel innovation wasn't purely scientific; it was also fueled by critical thinking and creative brainstorming. This fact persuades me that the way forward will take creative intelligence and design from all of us, using a vast array of skills, techniques, and areas of interest. We all can and ought to contribute to doing that.

Literature, fictional and nonfictional alike, has always been a crucial part of this reimagining process, because for much of human history we did not have the scientific tools now at our disposal. Even before Defoe, plague was often invoked in literature as a device to reveal the already morally diseased parts of society that were accepted as the status quo. Consider how widespread homelessness has now become a public health issue, or that minorities are suffering from COVID-19 at much higher rates than America's white population—in fact, zip codes can be used as one means of assessing COVID-19 risk. The homeless population has been problematically treated as expendable for decades, and their very existence has been criminalized as we outsource their management to police who are ill-equipped to handle such systemic social concerns. Similarly, economically disadvantaged communities have suffered from geographically based health inequities for decades, encountering as they do greater rates of dumping and pollution in their neighborhoods. To repeat: like the issue of underpaid grocery employees, im/migrant farm workers, or other people who cannot afford *not* to work, these problems are not new. They were simply more convenient for many of us to ignore before they became a public health issue. Like the Ghost of Christmas Future, the pandemic itself may very well be the grim reaper pointing at our existing sins while simultaneously shining a light on a new pathway for us—one in which we rethink our own privilege and reconsider who is essential, what that essential status means, whether the truly essential workers are paid as such, and so forth. The novel coronavirus, a tiny microscopic particle, has inarguably realigned the means by which we measure who and what jobs are essential. Addressing these social justice issues—keeping the human world in humoral balance—also enables us to achieve the goals of keeping the economy stable and working. Fail to pay grocery workers enough to incentivize their continued work under hazardous conditions? Well, then we all might go hungry.

It almost goes without saying that the major cost-benefit analysis at play when it comes to reopening businesses is the risk to human life. As I said in the introduction, this is not a health recommendation book, nor will I attempt to debate which scientific findings have been more valid than others. To do so would only add to the exhausting hum of voices arguing already. My aim is rather to explain how our thinking about these numbers and data is shaped, and how that thinking then shapes us and our concerns about businesses, such as the cost of economic movement to human life. Perhaps then we can reframe how we're asking and answering these questions and hopefully move these debates forward.

In another life, I was essentially a statistician. More specifically, I was in a clinical psychology PhD program specializing in psychometrics, which is the development of statistical measures of different psychological and cognitive phenomena (think IQ or personality tests). I didn't stay in the program long, having quickly realized my calling was elsewhere, but let me tell you—my twenty-two-year-old self was insatiable for statistics. It feels like something from another lifetime, but I recall literally thinking at one time that if we just got the math right, we truly could create a utopia on earth using statistics and actuarial tables. (Actuarial tables are statistical charts of liability and risk factors, among other things, that insurance companies use to determine their rates.) I can't fully express to you how much I loved statistics and their study and application. So, I hope you'll let this brief introduction serve as my résumé when I tell you that

LESSON 6:
Statistics are our frenemies, so no, risk elimination isn't actually possible.

"Death, death, death!"[11] H.F. looked up from his walk to his brother's house in Coleman Street. The sound had come from a window above him, where a woman leaned out the window and . . . just shrieked. Though her screams strike the narrator with "horror and a chillness in [his] very blood," he looks around, and the only answer to her grief is silence. No one walks the streets much during the plague in *A Journal*,

---

11   Ibid., 81.

where London has become a silent tomb of death. The only exception is when someone emerges in a frenzied panic to rave in grief or fear. H.F. remarks that no one so much as opened a window to see what the woman was screaming about because "people had no curiosity now in any case, nor could anybody help one another."[12] H.F., too, silently walked on, surrounded by a similar silence until the next person runs past him screaming hysterically.

To be fair, this moment has nothing to do with statistics, but it does have everything to do with ping-ponging from the extreme of silence and unfeeling to the other extreme of hysteria and grief. Statistics have a tendency to do the same thing to us, particularly when they track mass trauma and death. Yet they are a necessary evil, as we can't scientifically assess trauma and death without them. They are our frenemies.

In other words, we need them because they help us collect and understand data in so many ways, but humans—and our reactions to human issues—simply can never be fully reduced to numbers. I don't mean this as the wistful emotional statement it might sound like. I mean that cognitively, we have a lot of proof (from statistics, ironically) that humans are terrible at finding holistic, comprehensive meaning in statistical data. In short, our gut reactions to the statistics we encounter in media are often not reasonable deductions from that data.

Media saturation with people-as-death-statistics far too easily numbs us to the sheer enormity of the losses these numbers represent. The numbers, for all their necessity and value, dehumanize the very humans they signify. That's the point of an actuarial table, after all— to reduce humans to data points we can analyze to better understand the humans they represent. But when we've been exposed to human death as mere numbers for weeks or months, as with the COVID-19

---

12 Ibid.

epidemic, we become accustomed to thinking of the numbers as numbers, not as lives. We can't possibly imagine 500,000 deaths. In fact, the need for human scaling is a critical factor in studies of what makes scientific communication useful and understandable.[13] Five hundred thousand is not a number at a human scale. We cannot imagine 500,000 unique, "never to be had again" lives.[14] They become meaningless symbols, disconnected from the forever-lost, rich human lives they represent. Psychologists describe this effect as "psychic numbing," and psychologist Paul Slovic explains it bluntly: "The more who die, the less we care."[15] If that statement seems rather extreme, he expands on it in pretty persuasive terms, explaining that "the difference between zero people at risk and one is huge. But if I told you that there were eighty-seven people in danger in some situation, and then I told you that, oh no, there's eighty-eight, you won't feel any different; [but] a single individual, unlike a group, is viewed as a psychologically coherent unit. This leads to more extensive processing of information and stronger impressions about individuals than about groups."[16]

---

13 Michael F. Dahlstrom, "Using Narratives and Storytelling to Communicate Science with Nonexpert Audiences," *Proceedings of the National Academy of Sciences* 111 (2014): 13614–20, doi:10.1073/pnas.1320645111.

14 Kari Nixon, "Grieving our Collective Loss, One Stitch at a Time," *YES!*, May 1, 2020, www.yesmagazine.org/opinion/2020/05/01/coronavirus-death-grief/.

15 Andrew Dorn, "Here's Why People Care Less as More People Die and How That Impacts the COVID-19 Pandemic," ABC 10 Portland, August 11, 2020, www.abc10.com/article/tech/science/psychic-numbing-why-we-stop-caring/283-35da22bd-0fc3-4880-909b-8b3c4053476a. In this article, Dorn discusses an interview with Slovic, in which Slovic explains his article (see the next footnote) in lay terms.

16 Ibid.; Paul Slovic and Daniel Västfjäll, "The More Who Die, the Less We Care: Psychic Numbing and Genocide," in *Imagining Human Rights*, eds. Susanne Kaul and David Kim (Berlin: De Gruyter, 2015), 55–68.

―――

H.F. trudged through his neighborhood toward his house after another dismal day of death in London. His blood ran cold as he passed a house near his with the dead cart outside. *The maid, and an apprentice,* he heard the cartsmen say. H.F. was glued to the spot with horror, but he simultaneously wanted to run—run far, far away from the overreaching hand of death, away from the infection that had now reached his neighbor's home.

As he walked toward his shop the next morning, a Tuesday, he caught wind that two of the family's children and another apprentice had taken ill. His walk to and from his shop began to be punctuated by this one family's personal death statistics. How ironic, he thought, that he, who was so carefully tracking citywide and national death tolls, would now be so preoccupied by a family of ten and their small, little, personal griefs set against a backdrop of yawning, all-consuming death. By the week's end, however, there were no more small griefs to track; the entire household had died.[17]

―――

But something important happens to the psychically numbed mind when it is inevitably confronted with the fleshy human weight of death—that is, when a friend of a friend, an acquaintance, or a loved one dies of COVID-19, or any other deadly virus for that matter. It is my belief that our preexisting desensitization primes us to overreact at this point in the other direction. Like ostriches who had our heads (unintentionally) buried in the sand—full of two-dimensional numbers that can't possibly encapsulate the fullness of even one human life— we then get smacked in the head with the reality of death. Suddenly,

―――

17   Defoe, *Journal of the Plague Year,* 173–74.

from the mind-numbing insensibility of one million deaths, we see one death right in front of us, and as Slovic notes, we much more readily process and react to tragedy in the singular. From there, in my opinion, we go reeling into surprise and panic, and when we lose our emotional middle ground, we're also more subject to political extremities, too. For, as I will discuss more in **Lesson 12**, new and possibly distressing information that opposes our existing worldview tends to send us rushing to reaffirm the secure feeling of existing social bonds (such as like-minded politics in our personal echo chambers) and further causes us to simultaneously fight with anything that opposes it—a double whammy of synchronized fight-flight that quickly spirals out of control. A more toned-down version of this denial-panic cycle might look like hypervigilance alternating with vigilance fatigue, but the dynamic is similar, and their impacts, I think, are almost identical.[18]

Even as a historic disease scholar, up until 2020, I thought it was comical how much of Defoe's two books on plague consisted mostly of (often made-up) charts tracking death. It always seemed odd to me that a society blessed with some of the very first novels in their language—a genre we take for granted now—would use this form for rudimentary data-tracking of death charts—pages and pages of them, and many of them imaginary at that.

But today, I get it. Isn't this what so much of our life became once the COVID-19 pandemic began? Even if we're not seeking them out, our media content is bloated with death statistics. And on some level, we all seek this information at least now and then. We want to data-hoard, to see if the slow hand of death is coming for us next. We believe data is power, and of course it can be, but to some extent this

---

18 Dan M. Kahan, Ellen Peters, Maggie Wittlin, Paul Slovic, Lisa L. Ouellette, Donald Braman, and Gregory Mandel, "The Polarizing Impact of Science Literacy and Numeracy on Perceived Climate Change Risks," *Nature Climate Change* 2 (2012): 732–35.

		Of all Diseases.	Of the Plague.
	Aug. 8. to Aug. 15	5319	3880
	———— to 12	5668	4237
	———— to 29	7496	6102
From	Aug. 29. to Sept. 5	8252	6988
	———— to 12	7690	6544
	———— to 19	8297	7165
	———— to 30	6400	5533
	Sept. 27. to Oct. 3	5728	4929
	———— to 10	5068	4227
		59870	49705

Daniel Defoe, *A Journal of the Plague Year, as A History of the Plague in London* (Edinburgh: James Ballantyne and Co, 1810), p. 12.

belief has blinded us to the fact that data is fluid by its very nature. We want science to have ready-made answers, but we can lose trust in science when data changes what those answers are. So, another emotional pitfall that statistics can lead us into (along with our modern expectations from science and scientists, which I'll discuss in **Lesson 17**) is that they all too easily give us a false sense that data itself is static. This is a dangerous belief. Statistics are like a snapshot—a momentary attempt to capture in freeze-frame something that is always moving, always flowing (there's that word again, #sorrynotsorry), always already slipping away from our grasp. Of course, we don't think these things consciously. Intellectually, we know that statistics are just this sort of snapshot, but when we wonder why people scoff at or question scientific claims about COVID-19 that have reversed or shifted over time, the culprit is less people who are unwilling to buy into science than it is general social attitudes that treat statistics as concrete, stable factors instead of samples or slices of life at a given moment in time. The data itself changes as more is gathered and as people change. This does not mean that the data is necessarily faulty (although it of course could be), but that our expectations of data are.

We are hardly the first to hold data to such unrealistic standards. Such expectations date back to the Enlightenment—Defoe and Lady Montagu's time—when the scientific method and ideas like scientific objectivity were new and exciting. The public fascination with numbers and data as useful tools for understanding the world are in fact demonstrated by Defoe's preoccupation with them in *A Journal*. From at least that time onward, humanity has retained the sort of overreverence for statistical sampling that paradoxically dead-ends in outright science denial. Rather than engaging in arguments with individuals whom we see as "ignoring evidence," I think we'd get much further if we, as a global society, worked to destabilize Enlightenment notions of science as stable knowledge. What if we envisioned statistical sampling more like soil or water sampling, where small observations of small amounts of a whole gave us an idea about what the whole might be like at a specific moment in time? We'd never assume soil or water would be static—instead, we know that they change and, you guessed it, flow. If we could manage to avoid these two frenemy pitfalls of statistics that cause us to (1) ping-pong between the poles of desensitization and panic (or hyper- and then fatigued vigilance), and also to (2) unconsciously assume or expect data stability, we would, I think, readily arrive at the conclusion that risk elimination is impossible; instead, we're simply making choices about which risks we're taking at any given time. Perhaps this, too, is something we can learn from the profusion of death charts in *A Journal of the Plague Year*. The statistics in the book are so plentiful, they feel like they could almost be "played" like a flipbook. What was so strikingly odd to me when I first read the book over a decade ago now seems like a reasonably fair way to present data—fleeting glimpses rather than crystallized fact, glimpses that shift and change depending on how you contextualize them around narrative information.

Let's return to the three brothers, as Defoe does numerous times throughout his book. They're still in the midst of the scene I recounted earlier, which goes on for some time as the brothers attempt to determine what to do.

Thomas grimaced as he crossed his leg over the other, the old arthritic ache making itself known as he did so.

"Even if I'm not turned out of my lodging, there's no work now. Sometimes I think I'd be better off behind true prison bars—there's guaranteed meals, leastwise." John, always the most nervous of the three, raised his eyebrows.

"What can we do, then? I'll be turned out next week when my landlords go to the country, and I've no work, either. Maybe we should do the same—flee to the country." Richard growled, and Thomas translated his grumbled sentiment:

"We'll die if we do that; no one will even take our money for food, nor let us come into their towns, much less into their houses. They're scared we'll infect them, since we come from London."[19]

John jumped up, his nervous energy having been ignited into indignation. "I'll take the food if they refuse my money—they can't claim I stole it if I tried to pay, or perhaps I might leave the money near them, too, to prove I'm no thief."

Thomas stared at him, trying to envision a life on the road, a

---

19 Defoe, *Journal of the Plague Year*, 122–23. This last statement by Thomas is a direct quote from Defoe; the rest is adapted.

life of grifted meals instead of honest work, a life where he knew they might very well be spreading contagion to those who feared them. But even then, he knew that he and his brothers would pack up and go as John had described.

━━━━━

People have to eat, after all. And people will try to survive at all costs—the human race itself is a testament to that. And if your public health measures do not match with private needs, then private citizens will flout such recommendations or mandates to do what they believe they need to do to survive. So, while Defoe stands in support of public health, he simultaneously urges carefully calibrating public health recommendations—through an overhaul of society and the economy if necessary—to align them closely with private interests so that contagion is more effectively controlled *through* these public health measures. If Defoe's insistence on flow emphasizes one thing, it's this: people cannot simply seal up their houses entirely—they must at the very least open a window for grocery delivery. Completely avoiding our fellow humans in our neighborhood, then, is not a viable solution for Defoe. On a national level, he urges, in support of **Lesson 5**, that complete trade embargoes will backfire and cause uncontrolled smuggling (and thus plague exposure to a nation). Thus, xenophobic ideas about protecting a nation from foreign exposure entirely are also not viable. Both of these attempts at complete risk elimination are in fact dangerous solutions, causing economic stagnation and resulting in uncontrolled backwash of contagion (via quarantine escapees or smuggling) rather than balanced flow.

Visualize a pot with pressurized water being pumped into it at a stable rate. Say that pot springs a few leaks. You can imagine that as you plug up leak after leak in a pressurized system, ironically more and more pressure is directed at the remaining surface area of the pot, making new leaks inevitable. In fact, these new "leaks" will be more like geysers, as the pressure in the pot seeks ventilation. According to Defoe, we'd be much better off anticipating and allowing for the slow siphoning off of this pressure than allowing it to build and explode of its own accord, out of our control. Pretending we can just avoid the leaks is not only inaccurate, it's self-defeating. In other words, let me say it again: risk elimination is simply not possible. We can only choose *how* we encounter risk, and *which* risks we choose to confront. Defoe addresses this directly in his books. For instance, in *A Journal of the Plague Year* H.F. all but scoffs at his brother's notion that "the best preparation for the Plague [is] to run away from it."[20] He notes that almost anyone wealthy enough to flee the city did so (and we've seen this during the 2020 pandemic as well), but for Defoe this idea is as laughable as it sounds. We cannot opt out of the human race entirely (the only means of perfectly contagious risk elimination), and if we could, we'd find it a rather hollow victory. Instead, what Defoe advocates for, over and over again, is risk *mitigation*.

I believe that when the world went into quarantine in March 2020, the idea of flattening the curve was an important and necessary one—even a communal one, in spite of the fact that it isolated each of us. Even I, an infectious disease scholar whose job requires me to think deeply about existential fears of death and dying (I promise I'm tons of fun at parties, though), had been privileged enough that prior to the 2020 pandemic, I had never so much as contemplated the idea of hospitals in the Western world running out of resources. The curve had to be flattened. What I saw a few months into the 2020 lockdowns began to concern me, however. I watched many who had been alongside me, advocating for curve-flattening, now appear to inch the goalposts back. It was as though once the first world awoke to

---

20 Ibid., 9.

what had always been true—that infectious disease is still a threat—no amount of risk was tolerable, not even the risks we had always taken our entire lives. A December 2020 *LA Times* article noted that the "abstinence" approach we've been using in respect to contact and risk isn't working. As with promoting "safe sex," when it comes to pandemic guidelines, we need an approach of moderation and mitigation (or "harm reduction," as the article, and various public health specialists, terms it), not total elimination.[21] The latter simply isn't sustainable, and as Defoe and more recent commentators point out, it's possibly ineffective as well.

For most of our lives, we took risks with infectious disease that are simply highlighted now by the pandemic (in the same manner as systemic inequalities are, per **Lesson 5**). Some of these risks, such as not washing hands enough or not wearing masks (in the United States) when we were ill, we may decide never to take again—and that would be well and fine. But in essence these are still only risk mitigation tactics, not guarantees against risk entirely, and thinking of them as anything else, or trying to indulge in the delusion that they do guarantee perfect safety, has a number of disastrous consequences. Again, I will not propose to make specific health recommendations in this book, so what I'm saying here does not amount to a call to reopen society or to throw caution to the wind, or even an attempt to weigh in on whether the novel coronavirus is or is not more serious than the seasonal influenza. Instead, I'm making the claim, backed by my research in history and literature, psychological science studies, and my own personal understanding of human nature that (1) humans are pretty terrible at innate risk assessment, so we (2) use statistics to aid

---

21 Soumya Karlamangla, "Many Aren't Buying Public Officials' 'Stay-at-Home' Message. Experts Say There's a Better Way," *Los Angeles Times*, December 7, 2020, https://www.latimes.com/california/story/2020-12-07/coronavirus-stay-home -messaging-la-harm-reduction.

our understanding, but (3) said statistics only take us so far, because at the end of the day, they still rely on us as humans to assess the risks they may or may not highlight, and (4) humans are pretty terrible at risk assessment.

––––––––

Recall that statistics themselves can put us in a denial-panic cycle to begin with and encourage us to misunderstand data as static and unchanging. When this leads to a faulty belief (however subconscious) that risk elimination is possible, we can end up in a data war where opposing sides throw statistics and studies like bombs, some encouraging panic and fear and some encouraging denial. Neither is right, and neither is accurate, because both are extremist. Psychological studies (and common sense, really) show us that humans are even worse assessors of risk when we're in a state of fear—my colleague social psychology professor Patricia Bruininks, whom I'm lucky enough to also call a friend, explains this beautifully: "People in general are terrible at risk assessment, especially when in a state of fear. Fear and other anticipatory emotions lead us to focus on the possibility of something happening, not the probability. This is particularly true when what we fear is of great magnitude."[22]

She cites Loewenstein et al. for this information, as they acknowledge that while humans "evaluate risk cognitively," they "react to it emotionally," adding that "emotional reactions are sensitive to the vividness of associated imagery, proximity in time, and a variety of other variables."[23] So, for instance, seeing a loved one actually die from disease is likely going to drastically change how "risky" we

––––––––

22 Personal communication, August 18, 2020.

23 George F. Loewenstein, Elke W. Weber, Christopher K. Hsee, and Ned Welch, "Risk as Feelings," *Psychological Bulletin* 127 (2001): 267–86.

think getting a disease like COVID-19 is, even if the actual statistics about that risk haven't changed at all. Having seen a loved one die from a related disease fifty years ago, however, will probably affect our sense of this risk less—again, while the data itself hasn't budged. We can have all the data in the world, but it's still up to us humans to *react* to that data, and we tend to do so based on feelings more than facts. This is where the overreactive, panicked pendulum swing comes into play. From this overreactive, hypervigilant state, we begin to try to incorporate complete risk elimination and end up in a state of vigilance fatigue, which FDA director Scott Gottlieb noted was already happening in American society by early September 2020.[24] This all too readily encourages us to then swing back the other way— toward the safe feeling of denial, or even the defeatism of vigilance fatigue. Here is where the dehumanizing, hollow nature of statistics comes in. These two states fuel each other: our desire for complete risk elimination causes us to go into fight-or-flight mode, but this quickly results in fatigue and shutdown. We can't maintain panic and vigilance forever, after all. Neither of these states, of course, are productive, and they both, unfortunately, come from our all-too-human reactions to our frenemy statistics. For, in spite of all our data hoarding, we are emotional creatures. We can't extract that part of ourselves to somehow become purely logical beings, and believing this is possible only sets us up for failure.

---

24   Tony Czuczka and Yuegi Yang, "Virus Fatigue Is Risk as U.S. Heads into Fall, Ex-FDA Head Says," *Bloomberg*, September 6, 2020, www.bloombergquint.com /coronavirus-outbreak/virus-fatigue-is-risk-as-u-s-heads-into-fall-ex-fda-head -says.

My favorite part of Defoe's *Due Preparations for the Plague* is its subtitle: *as Well for Soul as Body*.[25] Whether you prefer to frame it in a secular or religious context, we are more than mere sacks of meat filled with fluid. To put it in a less disgusting manner (although that's the way I always phrase it for my students), we are not just bodies. We have minds and hearts (shout-out to my workplace, Whitworth University, where this is a major part of their motto). Many would argue that even animals, too, have feelings and emotional depth. Just as we cannot reduce ourselves to pure logic, it's also a fallacy to aim for an impossible sort of total risk elimination that protects only our body.

Say we could somehow fully avoid the risk of infectious disease. We'd have to board ourselves up in our homes, never see anyone, sanitize everything we touch according to intricate directions, and overcook all our food, while also likely limiting the range of foods we eat and nutrients we absorb. This sounds like a sad and hollow existence to me. In previous scholarly works, I have called this an "antibiotic life." *Antibiotic* means, quite literally, anti-life. For me, the life of body only is not one I would strive to pursue. But accepting a life full of "biotic" (or life-giving) experiences means we must also accept the risk that comes with such experiences. I don't want these statements to be misused by people who are making arguments about "life is risk" on Facebook or Twitter. Such arguments are generally weaponized toward extremist stances of reopening, with zero plan for risk mitigation. I may sound like a broken record here, but it's a broken record our society desperately needs if we are to push through the walls of our own

---

25 Though it's nonfiction, *Due Preparations* ironically has fewer statistical charts of mortality and epidemiological spread than *A Journal*, with more of its data discussed mid-paragraph instead of being set aside in a table. About half of *Due Preparations* is written in the form of a conversation between different people, which is again somewhat ironic considering that it's categorized as "nonfiction."

deafening echo chambers. There is a middle ground, one in which we find ways to minimize or decrease risks for all *while* maintaining the life-giving parts of emotional interaction that make us human. We can use social structures that encourage businesses to keep thriving (and thus keep *us* thriving) *while* making their goods and services accessible for all. Nothing in life is truly either/or, and our current circumstances are no exception.

There are all sorts of risks in life—psychological, emotional, and existential. For me, living an antibiotic life is an existential hazard of the extremist risk elimination, which our problematic relationship with statistics causes. There are long-term emotional effects of children having to stay hunkered down in abusive homes for long periods. There are psychological impacts of isolation and minimal human interaction. There are real impacts of overstating the need for "hygiene theater," as Derek Thompson phrased it in the *Atlantic*, for people who struggle with classic obsessive-compulsive disorder.[26] (Because of the Victorian sanitary movement, which I'll discuss later, I prefer the term "sanitation theater," which I will use throughout this book.) But, you might ask, are these things worse than death? Perhaps you're a reader who thinks the answer is obviously not, but I've shown my hand already: I don't believe the issue is so simple. Rather, once more, I urge for a complexity of understanding and nuance that resists such unproductive binaries. What I mean here is that life preserved at any cost is not going to be the same form of life we tried to preserve in the first place.

Secondly, protecting some forms of life (biological) with futile aims at risk elimination leaves other parts of our robust lives (emotional, psychological, cognitive) by the wayside. After all, why do we

---

26 Derek Thompson, "Hygiene Theater Is a Huge Waste of Time," *Atlantic*, July 27, 2020, https://www.theatlantic.com/ideas/archive/2020/07/scourge-hygiene -theater/614599/.

fear dying and grieve the death of loved ones? Not because we mourn the loss of their bodies or fear the loss of our own but because we miss *them* themselves, because we desire our own experiences, or fear unknown ones. The fear of epidemic and pandemic disease is, then, a fear of social and emotional losses. This must factor into our decision making just as much as infection prevention itself does. The fear of physical suffering plays a role, of course, but as I mentioned in the introduction, what we're really talking about when we talk about disease is people, not bodies. There is so much to protect besides bodies alone, for we humans are large, we contain multitudes. And for all his entrepreneurial energy, that is a statement that I think Mr. Defoe would wholeheartedly agree with me on.

3

LET'S STICK TOGETHER

How Cholera Shaped the Way
We Understand Community

===========

1832, 1848, *and* 1854

City of Westminster
September 1, 1854

Reverend Whitehead pulled at his collar with one finger, allowing the first hint of fall air to whisper between his skin and his clothing. His walk through the slum of St. Giles and its putrid smells led finally to the parish of his destination, St. James's, and he sucked in the fresh air with relief. This respectable working district was full of much more pleasant sights and sounds. It wasn't fancy by any means, but anything was preferable to St. Giles. As he approached the house in the Berwick Street district where he had been summoned, he mused at the stark differences between the two neighboring parishes.[1]

---

1 This narrative adapted from Henry Whitehead, "The Broad Street Pump: An Episode in the Cholera Epidemic of 1854," *Macmillan's Magazine*, December 1865, 113.

Fellow Victorian disease scholar (yes, there are more of us!) Pamela Gilbert has shaped a great deal of my thinking about Whitehead and his findings. In her book *Mapping the Victorian Social Body*, Gilbert explains that London society in Whitehead's time had long held that the two areas were foils—St. Giles a place of squalor, filth, and indecency, while St. James's boasted a palace and regularly hosted royal events.[2] Of course, St. James's also housed many working-class residents as well, but the proximity of it to such finery gave it a greater symbolic sheen than St. Giles. It also made it easier to ignore the similarities between St. James's and St. Giles (as neighborhoods of the working poor) and instead focus on its differences (with St. James's seen as a respectable "West End" area). Gilbert explains that "upon examination, it is clear that the two parishes, in many neighborhoods not significantly economically at variance, were misread to be consistent with the myth" of their stark differences.[3] And the myth certainly persisted. That two such "different" districts should be in such close proximity was something Londoners often commented about, particularly as a useful case study in opposites where neighborhood infrastructure and demographics were concerned. No one living in London at the time could have suspected that a well of contaminated water in 1854 would topple this fantasy. As Gilbert neatly puts it, "The operation of such [myths] can perhaps best be seen when an event occurs which challenges it."[4] As it turns out, this moment in history is something of a wellspring of learning, showing that

---

2   I highly recommend her book. Her academic work is of the rare sort that's both down-to-earth and brilliant at the same time. Publication information can be found below.

3   Pamela Gilbert, *Mapping the Victorian Social Body* (Albany: SUNY University Press, 2004), 100.

4   Ibid., 84.

Lesson 7:   Community is contagion.

Lesson 8:   Contagion is community.

Lesson 9:   We are our brother's keeper.

———

Henry Whitehead snapped out of his reverie as he was shown into the house. His blood ran cold at what he saw. Four members of the household lay prostrate and deathly ill. In spite of their differing ages, they bore much in common at that moment: even the youngest of them had a sunken, aged appearance from dehydration, and they all had a horrifying blue skin tone from deoxygenation that Henry recognized all too well—indeed, he'd hoped he would never see it again. He watched, his heart in his throat, as the patients suffered the telltale painful spasms in their arms and legs. The air hung thick with the odors left by the unrelenting vomiting and diarrhea at the root of it all. There was no escaping the fact: the cholera was back in Britain.

Reverend Whitehead choked back his fear—*Could this be the start of the next epidemic? Would it be worse than the ones in 1832 and 1848?*—and then got to work comforting the patients in the home. Later, as he showed himself out of the house, he tried to shake off his feeling of dread. *Four cases did not an epidemic make*, he told himself. And besides, St. James's had never experienced an outbreak of cholera before, which many of his contemporaries would have attributed to the greater respectability and cleanliness of St. James's (more on that assumption later). Cholera, seen (at the time) as a disease of filth, had always struck the dirtier, poorer St. Giles neighborhood. So perhaps this wasn't cholera at all. He wasn't a physician—what did he know? His panic was probably misguided. As he rounded the corner, enjoying the fresh air, a welcome respite after the stench of the sickroom, he smiled as he saw the faces of two of his colleagues in the church. A good chat with friends was just what he needed to shake off groundless fears and refocus his energies for the remaining duties of the day. As he approached within earshot, however, his greeting caught in his throat. Both the curate and the scripture reader looked like they'd seen a ghost. They stood close together, talking in hushed tones. As he approached, he learned that they *had* seen a ghost—the ghost of cholera coming back to haunt the British Isles. Like him, they had spent all morning at the bedsides of cholera patients in St. James's.

Whitehead looked around aghast, as if dread had turned him to stone. How was it that the slum of St. Giles had not been touched? How, with its broken windows and bedraggled children, was St. Giles the picture of health right now—or at least of non-cholera health? And how was respectable St. James's, where he had spent hours just yesterday and heard nothing of cholera, how was this same St. James's in Westminster suddenly home to more victims than he could count? In fact, he realized, he was late to attend to the next parishioner's home. He said a hurried goodbye to his friends and walked on, dismayed to learn upon his arrival that this home, too, had asked him there to comfort the family through a cholera case. In fact, Reverend Whitehead would spend the rest of the day comforting sufferers in St. James's, and even eleven years later, he would recount somberly that only one of those he visited survived.

———

In just ten days, the 1854 St. James's cholera onslaught took seven hundred lives within a 250-yard radius, according to Whitehead's estimate. (John Snow, who I'll introduce to you in just a moment, thought it was somewhere more in the realm of five hundred people.) That's seven hundred deaths in an area about the size of two football fields. Apparently uncertain his readers would be able to comprehend the magnitude of so many deaths in such a small area (remember that human scaling issue from **Lesson 6**?), Whitehead added the following explanation: out of a set of forty-five adjacent homes in the district, forty-one lost at least one person to cholera. Imagine that—consider your neighborhood or subdivision and try to imagine *every* home losing a loved one in a week and a half. Ten days. The very idea is pretty staggering. Cholera was rapid and merciless, often killing patients within twenty-four hours of the first experience of symptoms.

We now know that cholera, like many gastrointestinal (GI) bugs, is transmitted via a fecal-oral route, which is about as gross as it sounds. This essentially means that when people come down with a GI bug, they shed bacterial particles in their fecal matter. Some bugs, like the highly contagious norovirus, are even believed to develop specific tricks such as slowing down a patient's digestion, which effectively increases the volume of explosive diarrhea, allowing the virus to infect more people widely and rapidly. If another person unwittingly touches a surface on which infected fecal matter has landed (often invisibly) and then eats or touches their mouth, they're infected, too. Of course, in the early to mid-1800s the means of cholera transmission was still a mystery—very, very few diseases would be definitively seen as contagious until the 1880s—and this made its spread even easier. There were no widely known protocols about handling soiled linens very carefully, and the trademark "rice water" colored diarrhea of cholera victims made it difficult to discern what exactly had been soiled, meaning that even if one had instinctively wanted to avoid touching contaminated items, doing so would have been very difficult.[5] Thus,

---

5 Pamela Gilbert, "On Cholera in Nineteenth-Century England," *BRANCH: Britain, Representation and Nineteenth-Century History*, May 2012, ed. Dino Franco Felluga, extension of *Romanticism and Victorianism on the Net*, www.branchcollective.org /?ps_articles=pamela-k-gilbert-on-cholera-in-nineteenth-century-england.

from cholera's first appearance in Sunderland in 1831, it ravaged a country that had never before encountered anything like it.

There was definitely something horrifying in the first appearance of cholera in England. As we know from the novel coronavirus, diseases we don't understand and have never seen before are simply more terrifying than things we're used to. We have no collective wisdom about how to handle them. Of course, folks in Britain had seen diarrheal illnesses before, but they'd never seen anything like cholera, which is visually horrifying. It systematically turns its victims into explosive flesh vessels primed for viral spread through bodily effusions. Along the way, it leaves its victims positively ghastly looking as they career rapidly toward death. After this initial appearance in the 1830s, cholera reappeared approximately every ten years in the nation, and so, by the 1854 outbreak, the horror of the unfamiliar was waning somewhat. What made this outbreak special, though, is that it would upend long-held Victorian notions about epidemiology, and from there it would go on to change everything Victorians thought they knew about society and their connections to their fellow man.

In a world still decades away from widespread acceptance of germ theory and its microscopic proof of disease-causing organisms (more about that in chapter 5), most Victorians believed that the vast majority of diseases were caused by filth. In the minds of most people living in the 1830s, therefore, cleanliness was less akin to godliness than to healthiness. As you might readily imagine, cleanliness was of course vastly easier for those who could afford servants than it would have been for, say, overworked factory laborers. Thus, for the Victorians, the connection between filth and disease easily became a one-to-one relationship between class and disease, with the lower classes thought to be contaminated essentially by virtue of their poverty. Although many histories of the 1854 outbreak today describe St. James's as a well-known slum (and Gilbert acknowledges that it was), the broader cultural myth of St. James's as a place of royal finery nevertheless influenced how contemporary Londoners saw the space, and the outbreak of a disease of filth in this area jarred their expectations about how the world was supposed to work. In essence, the 1854 cholera outbreak that decimated the respectable-seeming neighborhood of St. James's forced Victorians to reevaluate all they thought they knew about disease and society.

It was after this outbreak that a doctor named John Snow, who had been formulating his hypothesis about a waterborne source of cholera for some years, would famously crack the case. Today he is often known as one of the founding fathers of epidemiology. Like another epidemiological innovator a decade later, Ignaz Semmelweis (more on him in the next chapter), Snow would not truly develop anything like the germ theory of disease we know today. However, he did suspect that cholera might be waterborne. After carefully examining the locations of the infected patients and plotting them on a map, Snow discovered that a huge majority of cases centered around the Broad Street water pump. In fact, many families in the St. James's district went to the Broad Street pump instead of other, nearer pumps, because the Broad Street pump was reputed to be the "purest" source of water in the neighborhood, particularly in comparison to their own homes' admittedly foul cisterns. Ironically, these families who went out of their way to attain what they thought was cleaner water instead unwittingly consumed water tainted with cholera.

Medical historians endlessly debate where the myth of John Snow's sudden revelation ends and where the reality of his prior years of cholera research begins, and to what extent he made the data in 1854 fit his existing hypothesis. In particular, Gilbert points out that Snow's data could easily have supported the earlier idea that filth, class, and disease were correlated, were he to have applied clear demographic evidence (which was available at the time) indicating that the Golden Square area of St. James's (where the outbreak was centered) was not very much different in socioeconomic status than St. Giles. Instead, for most people, his data supported a belief in St. Giles and St. James's as opposites—it used a medical model to explain *away* the fact that a disease of filth had shockingly appeared in a respectable district: water doesn't obey boundaries, and contaminated water from local cesspools had seeped into the Broad Street pump of its own accord. I find Gilbert's reading of the incident incredibly compelling, because in my research, the historic "great men of science" are always part legend, part reality, meant to serve a variety of social purposes beyond mere historical "fact." For his part, although Reverend Whitehead was initially an opponent of Snow's, he ultimately came to agree with him after surveying residents of the area and questioning them about their water usage and health history. Regardless of the motivations for and reasoning behind his revelation, however, when John Snow pinpointed the Broad Street pump and had the handle of the pump removed, he made several things clear to society that we ought to take away as we confront COVID-19 and any future epidemics:

LESSON 7:
Community is contagion.

I'd be willing to bet money that before COVID-19, only a small minority of people regularly thought about the fact that literally every time we're around another human, we're sharing breath, skin cells, and, yes, a microbiome of helpful and harmful microorganisms. While contagious disease is evidence enough that this connection is often dangerous or even deadly, most of the time, I find it wondrous. Particularly in America, we're raised to believe that we sink and swim of our own volition. We're trained early on to be islands unto ourselves, to resist the urge to call upon—or, god forbid, rely upon—the community around us. I love the study of disease with a ferocity for this very reason—it calls our bluff about all of that. We are all connected. Down to our very cells, we are a community and microbes make it so. This bond is of course scary in some ways, but isn't it also beautiful? We aren't alone—we're part of a vast, intricate, ancient, multispecies community that connects us like invisible gossamer strands running among us all. Priscilla Wald, whom I mentioned in chapter 1, puts it this way: "Communicability configur[es] community," and we could equally say that community *confers* communicability.[6] Without us, of course, human diseases couldn't thrive (as microbiological organisms, that is). We are, oddly, a necessity to their existence, and so even though we consider them our enemy, we are nevertheless intertwined in their livelihoods, too.

A case study from the 1832 Sunderland outbreak—historically considered the first recognized appearance of cholera on British soil—will make humans' interwoven destinies clear in another way. This Sunderland case study begins with Mr. Embleton, a surgeon in Sunderland who treated a great number of sick cholera patients. He quickly caught the disease and died.

Sunderland, England
December 1831

Even in the midst of her grief, his mother, Mrs. Embleton, had enough of the no-nonsense rural British housewife in her bones to know that the housework stopped for no one. I can readily imagine her wiping

---

6 Priscilla Wald, *Contagious: Cultures, Carriers, and the Outbreak Narrative* (Durham, NC: Duke University Press, 2008), 12.

"sommat" from her eye with the corner of an apron as she met Louisa Woodhall, the family's washerwoman, at the door to hand over her dead son's clothes for washing. I can imagine the ache in her breast as she parted, even if temporarily, with some of the last things her darling son had touched.[7]

If this were a movie, the camera would jump-cut now to Louisa as she journeys to her lodgings in the upper part of town. She's a not-young-but-not-old woman of forty-two, and she carries the bundle of clothes with a faraway look in her eyes, as if she were hardly thinking of laundry at all. Economics might have forced her to expend her labors washing other people's clothes, but no one could dictate her mind's wanderings, and who could blame her for wanting more than laundry out of life, if only in her imaginings? Louisa put one hand on the doorframe as she reached her home, bracing the other hand on the small of her back and arching her lower spine, as if her body knew before she did that it would be overworked soon, hunched over the wash basin. From the moment she stepped inside, there was noise—noise of her young one scampering about her feet, noise of her husband asking about dinner, and the noise in her head as she looked around at all the washing she still had to do that day. She shoved the Embletons' laundry under the family bed, to be dealt with in its turn.

Another jump-cut would happen here, to show the three-person Woodhall family sleeping peacefully together in their bed. Now imagine each of the people you've just been introduced to—the doctor's mother, the washerwoman, her child, her husband—all falling like dominos, one lightly tapping the other and causing it to fall.[8] These

---

7   This incident adapted from one recounted in the *London Literary Gazette*, February 18, 1832, 98.

8   I've read over the document repeatedly, and it's somewhat unclear if Mrs. Embleton died before or after her son's clothes were sent to Louisa Woodhall, so I've taken a little bit of creative liberty with this particular depiction.

tiny connections, through the simple act of handing off clothing, killed four people. This is how cholera demonstrated to British society more than ever, and with stark visibility, that there were indeed connections between the serving classes and those whom they served.

LESSON 8:
Contagion is community.

What John Snow brought to the public eye is that we encounter this contagious connection everywhere we go, and with everything we touch, sometimes even with every word we speak. Because certain viruses and bacteria depend on humans as hosts for their survival as a species, we humans risk this connection anytime that we commune. In fact, the word *contagion* means "to touch together," and dates back to at least the fourteenth century, demonstrating an early awareness that human contact itself is always already a risk for contagion.[9] My own scholarly book, *Kept from All Contagion: Germ Theory, Disease, and the Dilemma of Human Contact*, addresses these two lessons in book-length form, but here I'll simply boil it down for you: all human contact contains some element of risk. Every time we come near another human, we risk contagious disease. This is simply a biological fact. Most of the time, we come out on the other end of this gamble okay, and I have argued in my previous book that to completely avoid contagious disease risk is to completely dissolve society altogether, each of us actually becoming what America has always told us we were: isolated islands, devoid of any social connection whatsoever. Humans need connection with other humans because we are fundamentally social creatures at our core. If we focus only on protecting our biological lives perfectly (which would mean isolated perfectly

9 Wald, *Contagious*, 12.

and forever), we lose an important part of the human condition that's found in community.

Do my previous arguments mean that I take issue with the global movements in 2020 to socially distance and self-quarantine? Absolutely not. There's a difference between hermetically sealing oneself off from all risk with a goal of saving oneself or one's own family only and temporarily "pausing" our daily interactions for the very purpose of preserving the global community that so fundamentally contributes to this social human condition. To me, and based on my own previous work, what we've done in 2020 is not a single-minded focus on biological life. For one, we know that most people will not acquire COVID-19 in a severe form, so these global self-quarantining movements are aimed outward, at protecting those around us, not necessarily our own selves in most cases. Secondly, we're doing what we're doing with the purpose of preventing a virus from totally wiping us out as a species. What we have done with our collective Quarantine Life is a public recognition that

LESSON 9:
We are our brother's keeper.

I don't care what religion or dogma you subscribe to, the phrase is a good and a useful one. If disease microbes demonstrate that we are all connected (and they most certainly do), then it's a biological fact that we all have a stake in one another's success. If only for selfish reasons, it behooves all of us to ensure the safety of all of us. This is in fact the guiding principle of the One Health approach, a collaborative, interdisciplinary initiative with branches located in many different national and global health organizations. One Health aims to demonstrate that our future health as a species is even wrapped up with microbial success and survival, along with that of animals and the environment.

Environmentalism, too, is concerned with this idea. To stick with the example of water: we can't survive without it, so the sustainability of water sources is important to our survival. This is simply a fact, regardless of our priorities. If we fail to prioritize sustainable clean water sources, we'll die, no matter our level of concern for all the other living things around us. There's no way around it. Of course, I personally hope that we would care about one another and other animal and environmental entities for reasons beyond our own self-interest. But self-interest is hopefully a motivator even for those who want to look askance at communitarian goals.

So when he pinpointed the local water pump as the source of St. James's outbreak, whether he intended this message or not, John Snow also revealed that we share in the fate of our global neighborhood. In this particular case, he demonstrated that disease connects us all, like the air—or water—we all share, but this idea can be extrapolated to a broader notion of human, animal, and environmental connectivity. Even should we attempt to distribute water in ways that align neatly with our own ideas of society (such as separate water pumps for separate neighborhoods), the natural environment refuses to mimic our imaginary social barriers. Water simply flows. In spite of all we can build to contain it, water, as with other natural elements such as fire, earth, wind, and so forth, can and will forge its own path, sometimes through the smallest portals imaginable. In the case of the Broad Street pump, an overly shallow well, its bricks were loose enough that water seeped through the mud and dirt into the well. The filth of one community became the hydration of another, demonstrating with gruesome literalness that we are all connected, no matter how much we'd like to believe otherwise. This lesson will be repeated throughout later chapters of this book, because I think it's one of the most vitally important things disease has to teach us.

Although William Farr used his skills to disagree with Snow until much after the latter's death, my favorite cholera map is Farr's. The circular representations of cholera across varying temperature ranges look like ink slowly spilling out of a jar, and the images remind me of the slow and persistent flow of connection in community—often made visible through contagion—that so horrified Britons in the 1850s. The patterns are mesmerizing, illustrated in the original in colors of red, yellow, and black to demonstrate shifting cholera patterns in different times and temperatures. The images seem almost mobile, and I imagine the tricolored ink spill gradually growing in diameter, a slow but persistent menace. It's jarring to realize that this "ink" represents human lives, so much human life force ebbing away outside its corporeal boundaries, just as the colors exceed the lines of William Farr's circle graphs. Although Farr spent much of his life believing cholera was spread by foul odors from sewage, his illustrations still insist on the inevitable connection of all human life, in much the same way that Snow's discoveries about water did.

In some ways the Victorians speak for themselves quite eloquently on the issue, so I'll let their words close this chapter. These sentiments are from the same author recounting the trails of epidemiological connection in Sunderland described earlier. He reflected that "when there was sea there was communication, and when there was land [cholera] marked its progress so distinctly, that the line of its course has been traced upon a map, as if the personification of a pestilence has been traveling over the different countries of Europe and Asia, leaving the mark of a finger behind him."[10]

Ironically enough, fingers as communicable human connection would come to characterize the medical moment covered in our next chapter.

---

10   *London Literary Gazette*, February 18, 1832, 97.

4

WASH YOUR HANDS

Sanitation Campaigns throughout History

---

ca. 1845-1875

Vienna
1847

Ignaz sat grumbling at his desk, frustrated and antsy. The day had been long, his feet ached from his hospital rounds, and now he was finally at home, but he couldn't relax. His mind hummed with a frenetic energy that he knew from experience wouldn't stop until he could make sense of the conundrum that was preoccupying him.

He'd been appointed to Vienna General Hospital a few years before in 1844, and while obstetrics had never been his first choice for a specialty (he'd applied for both pathology and clinical medicine prior), he'd accepted the position cheerfully enough, ready to do good work for the women served by the hospital. And yet. *And yet, and yet, and yet.* His mind hummed on, turning over a problem he hadn't yet even been able to define. He couldn't quite put his finger on it, but something was very wrong in his hospital.

At least, this is how I envision Ignaz Semmelweis on the evenings and days that would precede his greatest act, because as a writer and a professor, I've felt this all-consuming "mind hum" myself. Unable to let the nagging problem go, Semmelweis would eventually unravel an undiscovered taint at the heart of his hospital, a revelation that would ultimately change the medical field forever. When I'm trying to figure out how to start a new book chapter—even this one, actually—or when I'm mulling over two seemingly contradictory ideas in my research to discover how they fit together, I can almost feel my mind tangibly ensnare the idea, as if with squid-like tentacles, feeling out all its parts, turning it over with octopus arms, exploring each nook and cranny of the problem, and absolutely refusing to let it go. Parts of my mind turn away, maybe momentarily looking over here or dealing with that interruption over there. But always, always, at least one tiny sucker stays attached to the problem in the background, worrying away at it out of sight, while to the rest of the world I appear to be answering their questions, fulfilling my duties. Of course, like so many of the anecdotes in this book, I can't know that's how Semmelweis felt, but I'm pretty confident in my assessment of this one, because as a fellow academic, I know this for certain: what Semmelweis discovered, what he had worried away at so long, at the end of that day, was solved because he couldn't. Let. It. Go. No matter what happened.

And once Ignaz discovered what he discovered, he refused to let anyone ignore him, consequences be damned. And there were consequences. He would be reviled by many of his fellow physicians for his revelations. He would even lose his job, and he would eventually die in ignominy in a mental institution, perhaps because of the Cassandra-esque curse of knowing a truth that no one would believe. Historians debate whether or not his institutionalization can really be attributed to the controversy that his discoveries incited, and at a distance of 150 years, we can never fully know what happened in his own mind at the end of his life, or why.[1] But the facts remain: Semmelweis, whose name is famous today, was hardly celebrated in his own day—far from it.

———

When he made his great discovery, though, Semmelweis was at the height of his career and primed for success and adulation. Still at his desk, he gazed into the middle distance, his mind turning over and over his experiences at the hospital. He ignored his dinner growing cold. He couldn't let this go. He had seen enough to know something wasn't right; he just didn't know what. He did know this, though: hospitals were supposed to help people. So why were all the women in Vienna General Hospital dying?

He would later recount, "Everything was uncertain, everything was inexplicable, only the enormous number of deaths was an indubitable fact."[2] One tentacle turned the problem over and over, moving a cell here, adjusting a theory there. He knew for a fact that he was doing all he could—all medical science could do—to help the pregnant women who gave birth in his hospital, and he assumed that his fellow physicians were as well. He tapped a finger on his desk in a rhythm that bespoke energized frustration.

A finger.

---

1 Likewise, we do not have a reason in writing as to why Semmelweis's medical appointment wasn't renewed in the midst of the controversy over his findings; historians must draw their own conclusions. Mine is that his discovery certainly played a role.

2 Ignaz Semmelweis, *The Etiology, the Concept, and the Prophylaxis of Childbed Fever*, trans. Frank Murphy, ed. Sherwin B. Nuland (Birmingham, UK: Classics of Medicine Library, 1981), 390.

His mind raced back to the dreadful day Jakob cut his finger. He was, in his own words, "totally shattered" by his friend and colleague's death. Jakob Kolletschka had been assisting his class with an autopsy, when a student accidentally sliced Jakob's finger with the scalpel. He had died of sepsis days later, with symptoms that looked all too familiar to the women on Ignaz's ward. *Could there . . .* A mind-tentacle gently turned over a whisper of a connection, considering. Was there a chance the scalpel had transferred something from the dead body's viscera into his friend's own body when it cut into his skin? "Day and night this picture of Kolletschka's disease pursued me," he would later recount.[3] I imagine Semmelweis's mind churning faster and faster, fitting the pieces of the puzzle into place with increasing rapidity as disparate observations coalesced into a clear theory. Suddenly, there was a pit in his stomach, and the inkstand in front of him swam before his eyes. He would later recount his horror at what he had realized. "God only knows," he would later write, "the number of women whom *I* have consigned prematurely to the grave."[4]

After he made this emotional connection, the theory that he translated onto paper was rigorous, systematic, and exhaustive. Semmelweis amassed enormous amounts of data based on his theory that something contagious was running through these hospitals, decimating families at their core by killing mothers shortly after childbirth. He carefully tracked maternal death rates across the hospital and noticed that women who gave birth in the ward presided over by doctors and medical students had higher death rates than women on the ward presided over by midwives. And not just a bit higher—it

3 Ibid., 391.

4 Quoted in William J. Sinclair, *Semmelweis: His Life and Doctrine: A Chapter in the History of Medicine* (Manchester, UK: Manchester University Press, 1909), 56; emphasis added.

was sixty in one ward and close to eight hundred in another. To put that in statistical terms, almost 1,000 percent more. He then collected mountains of data that meticulously compared the death rates in these two wards. Impressively, for an era still relatively new to detailed statistical research methodologies, Semmelweis essentially used the midwife ward as a control group against which to compare the actions of doctors. Using this analytical method, he was able to discount several other prevailing theories for the rampant maternal death in the doctors' ward. (Popular explanations at the time included foul airs that wafted between wards, dirty linens, and contaminated food, none of which could still be argued after Semmelweis collected his data, since both wards received all the same air, laundry, and food.) And after Jakob's death, he had a hunch. Midwives, after all, did not perform autopsies. As he pondered this in light of his data, he became certain that contaminating particles from sick, dead, and dying bodies were transmitted throughout the wards by doctors' hands.

The secret taint plaguing Vienna General Hospital was simply that— unwashed hands. In hospitals where doctors went from one childbirth to the next, sometimes stopping at an autopsy in between, infection (in this case Group A streptococcus, the same infection that causes strep throat) spread rapidly. Previously known by women as "childbed fever" and by medical professionals as "puerperal fever," the infection itself was not new. Indeed, it had long been considered a common hazard of childbearing. A well-known French proverb makes this clear: "Heaven stays open nine days for the mother in childbed."[5] Thus,

---

5 Quoted in Edward Shorter, *A History of Women's Bodies* (New York: Basic Books, 1982), 104.

while childbed fever was a known risk of childbirth that generally struck mothers (as the saying indicates) within a week after birth, it was Semmelweis's specific investigations that proved that doctors, who increasingly presided over the birth rooms where midwives had once reigned, might be the precise reason maternal mortality rates were often quite high.[6] Unlike midwives, doctors didn't only preside over childbirth, particularly in hospitals. To the modern mind, this is, of course, a recipe for contagious catastrophe. However, it took figures like Semmelweis to make this fact as obvious as it is for us today. His tireless, often aggressive advocacy for evidence-based practices, and the backlash he faced in return, highlights several key lessons we can still make use of today. Namely:

Lesson 10: **We must find common ground, or it will find us.**

Lesson 11: **The political is personal . . . for all of us.**

Lesson 12: **How you say things matters as much as what you say.**

Now, the notion that individual, specific germs cause individual, specific diseases would not be widely accepted for some time, when Louis Pasteur and Robert Koch's research would take the world stage (more on that later), but today Semmelweis's work is recognized to have been critical in edging society closer to this understanding. It's important to emphasize, though, that his understanding of germs

---

6 Specifically, the data we have from sources outside of Semmelweis about mortality at this time show that while other death rates were declining, maternal death rates remained high, and maternal death from puerperal fever specifically was increasing; see Richard C. Wertz and Dorothy Wertz, *Lying-In: A History of Childbirth in America* (New Haven, CT: Yale University Press, 1989).

and contagion wouldn't have looked like our own. He could follow the pathways of death and connect the dots between them, but he wasn't concerned with developing microbiological understandings of the responsible pathogen. Regardless, he did realize some sort of contamination was occurring between the bodies of doctors and the bodies of the women they served. While his work was important for germ theory's later development, at the time, Semmelweis was as much, if not more, concerned with practical solutions to stop the death.

His research went unpublished for years, but the knowledge was circulated among doctors and spoken about at public lectures. Its message was clear: wash your hands. After amassing his data, Semmelweis felt confident enough that doctors themselves were infecting women that he asked them to do something that at the time was radical. He asked them to wash their hands. Specifically, he requested that they wash their hands in a chloride of lime solution for about five minutes, until the skin was slippery from the substance.

It may surprise readers to learn that many doctors were at first violently opposed to the idea. I've mentioned that Semmelweis ultimately lost his job over his suggestions, and beyond his immediate circle, physicians the world over published angry articles opposing Semmelweis's ideas (although some did, of course, support his suggestions). Many doctors thought that Semmelweis was endangering women by encouraging them to indulge in worry and thus begin to fear their doctors. Victorians certainly thought fear and worry in general were bad for the health (and modern science has in some ways supported the notion that chronic stress has physiological consequences), and they most certainly infantilized women by presuming that worry could be exceedingly dangerous for "the gentler sex." In some obvious ways, then, the debates about handwashing, beginning as they did in obstetrical wards, are very much linked to gender and sexuality norms of the time. (For more on this specific aspect of the topic, I recommend the related chapter in my academic book, *Kept from All Contagion*.)

It has usually surprised my students through the years to find that handwashing—something we take so much for granted today— has a history, and that history involved a great deal of skepticism— even outrage—in its early days. Semmelweis himself was incredulous at the angry responses to his theories. Yet in light of the COVID-19 pandemic, I may just have to start anticipating a change in my students' reactions, because we have now all globally witnessed opposition to masking (a similar protective process), particularly in the United States. So, what can Semmelweis's history tell us about why so many people have gotten so angry about something that, for some others of us, seems like such a small ask?

LESSON 10:
We must find common ground, or it will find us.

Perhaps you haven't personally bristled at being asked to wear a mask, but you have almost certainly witnessed someone who did. Because of these disagreements, I think it's urgently important that we attempt to find common ground with and comprehend the reasoning of (even if we vehemently disagree with) those who stand in opposition to us. Many contend that the United States today—and much of the rest of the world—is undergoing a marked experience of political and social polarization in general. The specific context of COVID-19 makes the threat of polarization even more dangerous, because infectious diseases are a uniting force by their very nature, whether we like it or not. They visibly, sometimes grotesquely, demonstrate to us that we are all connected, all interdependent. To believe otherwise in the face of a global pandemic like COVID is to live in a delusion, and I would strongly suggest that this particular delusion could get us all killed. We must find common ground, if even on small issues. For if we refuse to accept this reality of our common human connection to one another, which disease makes so clear, then infectious disease will make it very, very clear by killing us all and leaving us united in the grave. One way or another, then, the truth of our interconnectedness will out.

I know that some more liberally minded readers will wonder why exactly so many have bristled at mask-wearing. To understand this mindset, the simplest mental exercise is to find a parallel but different example. That is, think of something you've done that essentially exhibits the same behavior, but over a different issue. You're essentially depoliticizing the issue—lowering the stakes so you can analyze, like a disinterested anthropologist, the common human thinking in such behaviors on neutral grounds, so to speak. Because

LESSON 11:
The political is personal . . . for all of us.

Erase from your mind right now all the party-line politics you associate with this phrase. Bodies are the most personal thing any of us have. It is, literally, our "person." And whether it's a government mandate to wear masks or your annoying know-it-all coworker who tells you to wash your hands, we all bristle, at least a little bit, at being told what to do with our own body by some outside authority. Society in general may very well be thought of as a constant tension between individual wants, needs, and desires and the need to sacrifice or set those things aside for societal demands. Taxation is one example of this, jury duty is another, and going to the DMV to update our car's registration yet another. Probably most of us would prefer to have our tax dollars back in our pocket, but we cough up the money either because we recognize it serves some larger purpose or simply because we don't want to be penalized for not doing so. Even liberal folks have probably sighed once or twice when they get their first paycheck at a new job and realize what portion of "their" money never lands in their own pocket. The point here is this: no matter where you fall on the political spectrum, most of us have in fact felt this tension between what we would personally prefer if we lived in a vacuum and the concessions we make to live within society.

The reason I love to teach about the science and medicine of the 1800s is precisely because it gives us historical examples just familiar enough to be relatable to our modern experience, yet just defamiliarized enough to allow us—should we be willing—to apply that sense to our own world. This experience allows us to examine our own norms and expectations with the distance of an anthropologist, considering dispassionately how we would act if these expectations weren't "givens." For example, it's hard to imagine a world where handwashing was reviled. The perplexity of this case study to the modern mind helps us see that it wasn't about the handwashing at all; nor is it, of course, really about the mask. My training prompts me next to ask: What was it about, then? If it wasn't about the science (in this case, a stand-in for the political), it must have been about the personal. In this example, I see "the personal" as being about many things—being told what to do with our bodies, being seemingly blamed as a vector of disease, and/or personal inconvenience or discomfort. (While it may seem surprising that anyone could decry handwashing as uncomfortable in the way we have seen in the masking debates, Semmelweis himself was said to have stripped entire layers of skin off his hands through vigorous chloride-lime washings, so the parallel between mask discomforts and handwashing discomforts are indeed present.)

Because I find that my students are often too willing to believe that "silly Victorian" objections to things like handwashing were simply because people of the past were less informed than we are today, and because I see a streak of a similar assumption about the supposed ignorance of mask opponents, I encourage the reader to come up with other, modern-day parallels that fit this pattern. Find some issue where deep down, you hate doing what you're "supposed" to do. Do you get annoyed that you have to mow your grass because your homeowner's association (not you) cares about the uniformity of grass height? Do you occasionally speed when you're running really late? Do you sometimes grumble when you put the toilet seat back down after having been nagged to do so a hundred times? These things are all personal—they require some labor, effort, or self-restraint on the part of an individual—but they have nothing to do with that individual's personal needs or desires: therefore, they're political, too. If even one of these examples resonates with you—even just a little—then you have some personal insight into the very human tendency to balk at being ordered to do something for someone else's benefit. And if you happen to be a reader who readily adopted mask-wearing, this means you've also found your first glimpse into your opposition's thought process. This is the first step, in my view, toward productive debate. If we assume the other party is ignorant or malicious (and of course these things obviously may sometimes be true, but the assumption is unhelpful), we've already lost traction in pulling together and uniting against a virus that threatens us all. Which brings us to

LESSON 12:
How you say things matters as much as what you say.

I'll keep it real: Semmelweis was kind of a jerk about the handwashing thing. He not only aggressively attacked doctors who weren't washing their hands in spite of his evidence (which, fair) but he could also be haughty and self-righteous about being a savior of women himself. He once famously called one of his dissenters a "murderer" and a "participant in a massacre."[7] One scholar has described Semmelweis as the legacy of an "unsuccessful attempt to implement a patient safety initiative," arguing that his failure "remains as instructive as his great achievements."[8] The way we explain things matters, after all (**Lesson 6**). Along the same lines, how we *approach* people with our explanations also matters. We'll never know if Semmelweis would have won more people over if he had tried to . . . well, win them over instead of long-distance screaming at them in angry letters. But we can avoid his likely misstep when we approach public health recommendations today, such as the prominent masking debates.

Doctors had been debating the causes of puerperal fever for some time, and in some ways the subject was already polarizing. Oliver Wendell Holmes, who agreed with Semmelweis, recounted the story of a physician some decades prior who had carried the uterus of a woman who had died of puerperal fever with him in his pocket to show his students, not changing clothes between this and his next birth. This man, William Campbell, was known to be an anti-contagionist (though he later changed his views), and some historians believe Campbell did

---

7   Nuland, xxxv–xxxvii.

8   Andrew Stewardson and Didier Pittet, "Ignác Semmelweis—Celebrating a Flawed Pioneer of Patient Safety," *Lancet* 378, no. 9785 (2011): 23.

this to demonstrate that the uterus would not transmit disease to the next woman (it did; she died). This demonstrates just how heated these debates could get even before Semmelweis took the stage with his aggressive approach.[9]

Before I go on, I want to be crystal clear about my message here, because in far too many instances in human history, calls for civility have really been a strategy of maintaining control over groups who have less power than others. For instance, the 2020 racial protests and ensuing property damage were often met with criticisms against the

---

9 I have to admit that this has been one of my favorite historical moments ever, but in double- and triple-checking facts for this book, I've come to the conclusion that we can't be precisely sure of Campbell's motives for the uterus-pocket moment. He may simply have wanted to show the specimen to his students, and, disbelieving the contagion theory of puerperal fever, saw nothing wrong with stowing it in this manner. Being that Campbell was an avowed anti-contagionist, he may very well have done this to make a point. Nevertheless, as I mentioned in chapter 1, Victorians are very real people to me, although they're long dead, and I'm uncomfortable assigning motivation to Campbell's actions. Campbell himself wrote about the incident twice (which is where Holmes found the story), and in none of these three accounts does either man say *why* he did this, only that he did it. That suggests to me that there was likely no real reason for Campbell's choice—perhaps a cavalier disavowal of a possible theory, to his thinking, at best. It is, of course, possible that Campbell made this choice as a flagrant display of his own opinions regarding contagion, but in general I find that Victorians are fairly forthcoming about their motives. If such a motive was the purpose of the display, why not mention it? Particularly since, when Campbell retells these case studies, he does so from the perspective of having decided that puerperal fever is indeed contagious. Again, we can't know for sure, but the uterus-pocket story will live in my memory forever as the best historical narrative ever told. The sources I tracked down to explore this further are listed in the works cited.

unruly nature of said protests. This all too easily allowed detractors (that is, those who were unhappy about the property violence) to ignore or deny the veracity of the claims made by the protestors about the inherent human rights of Black people. I will never prevaricate about or hide my own political leanings, though in many instances I think they can be set aside for the purposes of finding common ground from which to move forward. This means that generally, I think my political opinions are irrelevant in most cases. But this moment calls for an exception: I vehemently believe Black lives matter, and I most definitely think focusing on the property damage of those protests is an insidious strategy that serves only to ignore the urgent needs of those protestors—the need to be treated humanely and as humans.

So, it will be clear by this statement that I do not intend what I'm about to say as a call for "niceness" when we communicate needs. I'm not calling for plain old "niceness." What I'm calling for is effectiveness. In the realm of social media, where most of us have a ready platform (and often readily engage in fights with opposing parties), it is here that I claim arguing about masks in particular, and health recommendations most generally, may go further if we don't personally see our opposition as an enemy.

———

I don't believe Semmelweis was intending to be "mean" or "nice." I believe he actually thought his fellow physicians were willfully ignoring his recommendations, and, if this is so, then Semmelweis's harsh words were unfortunately correct. However, while we can't know each and every individual physician's motivations, there were in fact many reasons that physicians were incredulous about or skeptical of Semmelweis's recommendations, aside from willful ignorance. For one, statistical science as we know it today was then in its infancy; ironically enough, using such innovative means of explaining his reasoning may have made it less believable than if he had relied on more well-known means of explanation. Secondly, Semmelweis didn't particularly care about developing a model to explain how his theory of contamination worked—such models would come about twenty years later (and will be covered in later chapters). In his mind, he had demonstrated that the effect of contamination existed and that it was preventable, and that should be enough. But as history would demonstrate, simply expecting his peers to understand a completely world-changing view of contamination and their own bodies using methods of proof that they weren't familiar with . . . well, it was a pretty weak strategy. As is evident by the CDC's vacillating messages on mask-wearing in early 2020, our problematic view of data and science as stable facts (**Lesson 6**) makes humans all too ready to balk when the fluidity of said data is revealed. The answer here isn't more disdain for supposed "science deniers" but a broader campaign of reframing how society as a whole views science. It's time to move beyond Enlightenment-era expectations.

Additionally, as I've said, in my research, I've found that it's a fairly common human reaction to resist being told what to do with your body. I think this is a critical consideration to keep in mind when discussing public health recommendations—whether you're a doctor, a policymaker, or just fighting with your mom's friend on Facebook. When dealing with the already thorny issue of public health recommendations, it's vitally important that we first cease to see our opposition as the enemy, and then consider from a position of empathy and understanding what may be the roadblocks to other people's acceptance of the data or recommendations we're promoting. Only *then* can we move on to changing opinions and behaviors in others.

Numerous studies on the communication of scientific information suggest that narrative is an important driver of comprehension and acceptance.[10] People don't just want facts or data; they want a story to demonstrate why it should matter—and the present book is no exception. I could have easily drafted this project as a dry critical-thinking textbook or a timeline-based history book. But would you have read this far in either of them? I've already hinted at the first rule of effective narrative: you can't tell a good story when you believe your audience is hostile, or when you're hostile to them. It therefore also holds true that you cannot assume that the audience can't understand you or isn't able to intellectually process your thesis. (Because seriously, have you ever seen that go well?) Broad generalizations rarely hold water, but I can't imagine any circumstance in which effective teaching takes place through a teacher who believes from the outset that their students are incapable of learning or unwilling to listen. Beyond this, however, I see far too many highly scientifically literate people assuming not only that those who disagree with them simply don't understand the data they're promoting but also that if they just keep repeating the data confidently, they'll eventually badger their opposition into submission. Which also doesn't usually go well; remember how that turned out for Semmelweis? He may have been right, but he wasn't particularly effective during his lifetime.

In stark opposition to this stance, scientific communication studies also tell us that scientific literacy has very little to do with *responses* to science. We might assume that the greater one's scientific literacy, the greater one's ability to comprehend and understand newly pre-

---

10 Dahlstrom (2014) is one such study, and so is Kahan et al. (2010) (both are cited in the previous chapters' footnotes). Another valuable study is Donald Braman, Dan M. Kahan, Ellen Peters, Maggie Wittlin, Paul Slovic, Lisa Larrimore Ouellette, and Gregory N. Mandel, "The Polarizing Impact of Science Literacy and Numeracy on Perceived Climate Change Risks," *Scholarly Commons, Nature Climate Change* 2 (2012): 732–35, http://scholarship.law.gwu.edu/faculty_publications/265.

sented scientific data. However, research demonstrates that, particularly when the topic is a polarizing one—and by now I hope it's clear that public health recommendations are polarizing by definition (**Lesson 2**)—greater scientific literacy surprisingly leads to a higher chance that the listener will simply double down on their previously held view.

It's simply impossible to deny that humans are social animals, and when faced with a new and uncertain situation, being presented with new and uncertain data doesn't encourage our agreement; instead, it motivates us to turn to the social bonds and groups that give us certainty and comfort.[11] We are *always* going to pick group acceptance over cold, hard facts, and only the more so when the cold, hard facts make us uneasy or highlight an inconvenient truth. But that does not mean we should ignore or abandon the facts. It means that it is misguided to believe that shouting the facts louder will persuade people—in fact, it may very well do the opposite. Instead, if we work toward finding common ground, toward realizing that we are all basically social creatures who need acceptance and belonging, that whether we like it or not, on some level we understand the desire not to wear masks (or not mow the lawn or not pay taxes, **Lesson 10**), then we will already have grasped **Lesson 11**. We will no longer be able to see our opponents as fundamentally different from us—as somehow more selfish, less loving, less human—and when that occurs, we will likely already be presenting our facts in a very different way to begin with (**Lesson 12**). In the next few chapters, we'll explore what these differences in presentation may need to look like to be effective, and we'll do this primarily by exploring what I see to be the historical factors that have shaped modern, Western attitudes toward death, disease, and risk.

---

11   Ibid.

5

GERMS, GERMS EVERYWHERE

How Discovering Bacteria Saved Humanity—
and How It Might Destroy Us

═══════

1875-1901

Imagine that the United States is preparing for an outbreak of
an unusual disease that is expected to kill 600 people. You're an
epidemiologist and you've been asked to choose between two dif-
ferent programs to combat the disease. The estimates about suc-
cess are exact. If you choose program A, 200 people will be saved.
If you choose program B, there is a ⅓ probability that 600 people
will be saved and a ⅔ probability that no one will be saved.
Which of the two programs would you favor?[1]

Everybody, stop! It's reflection time! Before you read further, stop
and decide which option you would pick. I'll go ahead and spoil just

─────────

1 Daniel Kahneman and Amos Tversky, "Prospect Theory: An Analysis of Decision Under Risk," *Econometrica* 47 (1979): 263–92, and adapted in Katy Milkman, "Take the Deal!" *Choiceology* (podcast), season 4 episode 4, October 2019.

one detail: this question was written in 1979, and obviously has nothing to do with COVID-19. But hey, as I tell all my students, you're now unfortunately an expert at living through this mess, so go ahead, make a choice. Explain your reasoning. Here, I'll even give you some lines to write on, because I am ever the professor giving homework:

_____

_____

_____

_____

_____

_____

Okay! Think quick—here's another one:

Now, imagine that the United States is preparing for an outbreak of an unusual disease that is expected to kill 600 people. You're an epidemiologist and you've been asked to choose between two different programs to combat the disease. The estimates about success are exact. If you choose program A, 400 people will die. If you choose program B there is a ⅓ probability that nobody will die, and a ⅔ probability that 600 people will die. Which of the two programs do you favor?

Same thing. Think, reflect, respond, go!

_____

_____

_____

_____

_____

Although the above scenarios conveniently deal with infectious disease, they are in fact an artifact from a 1970s behavioral finance study, and the lessons of this chapter are drawn as much from the lessons of economics as from the lessons of history, as people define their perceived success differently depending upon their reference point. This study, performed by Israeli psychologists Daniel Kahneman and Amos Tversky, demonstrated the existence of what is now called prospect theory. Their work showed that people routinely chose Plan A in the first scenario and Plan B in the second, even though the two scenarios are mathematically and probabilistically identical. As Katy Milkman of the podcast *Choiceology* explains it: "Our taste for risk changes when we think of the very same decision with a focus on losses instead of gains."[2] To put the matter more simply, what a silver medalist perceives as a loss (of first place), a bronze medalist sees as a win (of *not* fourth place), and we can apply this cognitive bias to all forms of decisions humans make.

But, no, I'm not about to walk you through zombie-apocalypse-style public health decision making using the Kahneman and Tversky study. Although the example they used in their research coincidentally and conveniently draws upon epidemiology to make its point, they used this example to demonstrate points about decision making more generally, and I will use it as well to draw larger, existential points about how we think about disease in relation to ourselves. These are:

Lesson 13:   It ain't whack-a-mole.

Lesson 14:   Ironically, the "medical revolution" has caused us to live in denial of death.

---

2   Milkman, "Take the Deal!"

Lesson 15:   Life is like ~~a box of chocolates~~—er, a garden.

The previous chapters focused on how disease informs the way we think about and communicate with others. In this chapter, we're going to approach the problem from a different angle and begin from an inward perspective. Disease can definitely teach us much about how we should and do interact with others. But evolving disease science over time has also shaped how we conceptualize our own identities, as well as the way *we* think about the communities we're a part of, communities that disease itself shapes and informs.

———

A lot of my clearest memories from my early childhood—when I was around six or seven—involve a deep sense of commingled guilt and horror about climate change. These memories are less than glamorous: I'm always kneeling in front of the console TV where I spent unquestioned amounts of time watching cartoons. The eighties and early nineties were a time of unmitigated consumption of many things that no one much questioned in mainstream society, and it is perhaps for this reason that it seems to also have been the era of PSAs, fueled by the reassuring ideas that "knowledge is power" and if citizens *know* something, they'll *do* something differently or better. This was the era of "This is your brain on drugs" and "I learned it by watching you!" This was the era when we believed circulation of media could fix anything, primarily because society was more and more engrossed in media to begin with. So, I was exposed to a litany of PSAs about litter, recycling, the ozone layer, and many other things I was barely able to wrap my head around. This was a lot for a seven-year-old.

Anyway, my point is this: global warming and the changing ozone layer had existed prior to these media campaigns. The temperatures were changing, and notable changes were occurring planetwide. But for most people, global warming *didn't exist* until it was named as such and circulated in our daily dose of media. It's kind of like Schröding-er's cat, in a way. It may or may not be there for some scientists and experts, but it doesn't really "exist" meaningfully until there's a word for it, and a global concept of what this means, how we impact it, and how the concept impacts us. When *that* happens, however, not only does the concept exist but it's liable to become a pervasive way that we think about the world.

Recall One Health. Such a concept couldn't really mean anything to us until we had already come to see our livelihood as intertwined with the health of our planet, which couldn't happen until we began to understand the concept of global warming. Once that happened, however, our relationships to our goods and foods were all going to continue to shift over time, as we saw our own role in the health of the planet itself. Germ theory did something like this, and I pause on this eighties-tastic example because in the previous two chapters specifically, I've done something repeatedly that may very well be con-fusing: I've presented to you a series of different men of science who discovered certain diseases were contagious, and yet I've told you over and over that these revelations were *not* the same thing as the germ theory of disease. You may be asking yourself by now, how was what Semmelweis and Snow discovered any different than this? Or, for that matter, how can we claim that before the 1880s society *wasn't* aware of the existence of contagious disease, if we can quite readily see (ahem, chapter 2) that people in Defoe's era feared the infected folks around them?

To some extent, the honest answer is that the difference is one of semantics, and I'll get to that in just a moment. The more prag-matic answer is that the development of germ theory is often overly simplified as the moment society learned that contagious disease ex-isted. That's just not true. Some diseases—think the plague of Defoe's day—were quite obviously infectious. Diseases with dermatological symptoms like smallpox very visibly marked the patient in a particular, identifiable way, and if readily identifiable diseases like this also had quick incubation periods (i.e., a person interacts with a smallpox patient and the next day discovers the same marks on his skin), the conclusion of contagion was obvious and had been accepted in regard to certain diseases for centuries. Such conclusions were harder to draw with diseases that had long incubation periods or less obvious external symptoms (more on this in **Lesson 25**), and so while germ theory did not introduce the concept of contagion entirely to society—far from it—it did present contagion more widely as the cause of *many*, or even most, diseases.

Germ theory was more than anything a model explaining *how* contagion happened, rather than introducing contagion as a concept altogether. It was brought into the public understanding by a handful of scientists in the 1880s who worked feverishly (excuse the pun) not only to prove that contagion existed but also to illustrate *how it worked*. The public understanding part is key, because germ theory had vast effects on collective understandings of identity and community (think **Lessons 7 and 8** magnified to an enormous power). This broad understanding of germ theory in the public was only possible because scientific advances were frequently published in newspapers and magazines (rather than specialized journals today), meaning that most of the reading public was very much aware of scientific advancements, debates, and discoveries. Even today, some of the most famous germ theory scientists' names are ones we're still familiar with. Louis Pasteur was famously able to cause disease in healthy organisms by injecting them with matter from other, infected creatures. Importantly, he observed that *the exact same* disease would occur in the second organism. If you've ever consumed pasteurized milk or juice (spoiler alert: you have), then you've heard Pasteur's name; he was made famous for a process that eliminates the microorganisms he studied. Joseph Lister also studied processes in surgical patients that convinced him the germ theory of disease was undeniable, and he implemented means of antiseptic techniques to curb mortality rates—his name is now used as the root word for the antiseptic mouthwash Listerine. Less memorialized in American culture but just as influential nonetheless is Robert Koch, who took Pasteur's work on disease and systematized it into a methodical process that could be assessed with null hypotheses using the scientific method.

Koch insisted that to properly "prove" the existence of specific disease-causing microbes, matter had to be extracted from an organism sick with a disease easily recognized by clinical symptoms (smallpox, measles, etc.). Next, this matter had to be cultured in a petri dish (Julius Petri was one of Koch's assistants) and identified clearly under a microscope. That is, the bacteria's morphology had to be drawn on paper or clearly explained by an observer. Then, this matter had to be extracted *from* the petri dish, injected into a second organism, and the same disease had to be observed in this second organism using the same clinical criteria seen in the first organism. *Then*—Koch was relentlessly scrupulous—an additional sample of matter had to be taken from the second, newly sick organism and cultured in a second petri dish. This petri dish had to demonstrate the growth of the same-looking particle seen in the original dish. Then and only then could someone scientifically proclaim they had discovered the disease-causing microbe for a given disease. (Sorry, PETA: many chickens and bunnies were harmed in the making of this science.)

Koch's Postulates—which he derived from these experiments—are still widely taught to biology students today. It was a combination of the work of these scientists (along with others, of course) that proved that not only are *most* diseases contagious but that each disease we see manifested in the human body is the result of a highly specific microbe that can be named and identified readily. Suddenly, people could *see* their enemies, if only under the microscope. More astounding, they could now see that their enemies were all around them—in the air, the water, and the soil. It became clear that humanity was forever swimming in a sea of bacteria.

———

Okay, so what?

If you find yourself asking this, you're a better critical thinker than you may be giving yourself credit for. For one, this knowledge is so second nature to us today, only 140 years later, that it can be hard to figure out what the big deal was. (In fact, "what's the big deal?" was the question that led me to write my entire dissertation and later my first academic book.) You see, before germ theory, most people believed noxious airs—miasma—caused disease, and that places with bad air, rather than people, were what harbored disease. In the final three chapters of this book, we will see in great detail exactly what the consequences are of seeing one's fellow humans as the site of disease, as well as the practical problems this outlook introduces for disease containment. For the time being, we'll address the conceptual differences rather than ethical consequences. After all, if miasma theory supposed that disease-causing elements moved from place to place in the air, and germ theory supposed that disease-causing elements moved from person to person on, say, coughs and sneezes (aka air), what's really the difference? I often find that my students have a bit of a case of "the emperor's new clothes" with this question, assuming they're missing some critical information when they don't see much of a difference between the two. And because you likely are wondering, I'll just come right out and say it: you're not missing anything—the differences in some ways are quite minimal.

Before the germ theory of disease took over, ideas about disease management were dominated by what was known as the sanitary movement. Such practices ruled during Snow and Farr's time in the early 1800s and essentially included keeping spaces clean, and on a broader level, keeping sewage contained and separate from eating and drinking spaces. These remained society's only tools even after germ theory emerged. If you find this a bit anticlimactic, considering we tout this as one of modern medicine's greatest breakthroughs, you're not alone: many, many scholars have noticed that germ theory did quite little to fundamentally alter how society handled disease. I recommend the work of Bruno Latour and David Barnes particularly to this end. Both men—and, frankly, common sense—demonstrate that the tools of combatting disease were in fact no different after germ theory emerged than they were before it. Barnes particularly notes that existing modes of sanitary hygiene were simply grafted onto the conceptual model of germ theory in this later period. That is, the same tools of hygiene were being used; their effectiveness was simply justified using a new theoretical model.

In her book *Membranes: Metaphors of Invasion in Nineteenth-Century Literature, Science, and Politics*, historian of science and English professor Laura Otis argues that the popularity of germ theory over miasma in the late 1800s had much more to do with issues of power, politics, and control than any other force. For instance, she notes that in contrast to earlier, Montagu-era fears about influence from foreign cultures in the form of vaccination, in this later period, Europeans sought to enact "offensive" tactics against diseases they saw as coming from the "Others" they colonized—logic backed by what they hailed as Western science.[3] Otis notes that microorganisms could have "easily been [seen] with Leeuwenhoek's lenses in the 1670s," but until people *wanted* or *needed* to observe them as microbial pathogens, they weren't classified as such.[4] I find these arguments incredibly convincing. All

---

3   Laura Otis, *Membranes: Metaphors of Invasion in Nineteenth-Century Literature, Science, and Politics* (Baltimore: Johns Hopkins University Press, 2000), 34, quoting Koch.

4   Ibid., 4, quoting Brian Ford, *Single Lens: The Story of the Simple Microscope* (New York: Harper Collins, 1985), 130.

in all, germ theory offered very little new in human observation or in practical explanations. In many ways, then, it makes sense to explain the sudden "discovery" of germ theory as a move based in power and authority more than anything else, and certainly we shouldn't see it as one that really changed human life at a practical level at all; sweeping, dusting, and good old soap and water were still man's best friend when it came to disease. Sure, a doctor could tell you that you had gotten cholera from contaminated linens that had *Vibrio cholera* on them, but that wouldn't lead to new treatments or cures anytime soon.

But I believe there is one important cultural change that widespread belief in germ theory *caused*, even if germ theory itself was a somewhat arbitrary development in science. And that was the quantifiable, concrete, and observable *enemy* in the form of the microbe.

———

Let's say you had just developed cholera symptoms. By the 1880s, your friendly neighborhood doctor could accurately give you this diagnosis and would be able to explain to you that you likely caught it via bacterial organisms from someone you were close to. Let's be real, though: you were still toast. The only difference is that you could now observe your death sentence more concretely, and to understand, as you died, that tiny living organisms had invaded your body and taken it over, and that your brother or your neighbor or maybe even your kids had infected you.

I think this moment must have felt less like a scientific revolution and more like a pretty raw deal. The new understanding of germ-based contamination didn't bring along with it any new cures. It just made people more precisely aware of how they would—or, more important, how they *could*—die. The closest thing to a revolution that germ theory brought about for society was simply this: the enemy had been identified, and that enemy was a living thing. But this brought a certain kind of hope, for better or worse: living things could be killed, and we humans are very good at killing. So, while antibiotics and the like were still decades away from existing, humans at least had a target. Medical humanities scholar Lorenzo Servitje's book *Medicine Is War: The Martial Metaphor in Victorian Literature and Culture* describes the use of militaristic language in relationship to disease, and I recommend it if you're looking to discover more on the topic; for my purposes here, however, what I want to focus on is less the idea of germs as a killable enemy and more on what the *mere possibility of conquest* over disease did to the human psyche as a whole.[5]

Remember the hypothetical situation that opened this chapter? Based on my research on the popularization of germ theory in the 1880s (which just so happens to be my niche-of-a-niche-of-a-niche specialty), I believe this is the moment when humans changed the reference point by which they thought about disease and death. In other words, the reference point by which humans gauged the success of their very existence shifted in this era. We were no longer the bronze medalist, glad to simply have a spot on the platform (i.e., somehow not dying from all the menacing diseases out there); we became silver-medal sad— the "not impressed" gymnast McKayla Maroney side-eying our losses (why did we ever get sick at all?) instead of our gains.

Before germ theory was widely adopted, every near miss from death was a victory (bronze medal, loud and proud over here!). Even though the development and popular acceptance of germ theory didn't bring along with it any cures, I'm convinced it dangled the carrot of cures (the gold!) in front of society. It made people believe cures could

5 Lorenzo Servitje, *Medicine Is War: The Martial Metaphor in Victorian Literature and Culture* (Albany: SUNY University Press, 2021).

be found, readily, if we could only figure out how to kill all the germs. *BAM!* Just like that, we were silver-medal sad. Every death now instantly became situated around a different reference point, because freedom from infectious disease at least *felt* possible, even if it wasn't. From then on, deaths were seen more as losses that *should* have been preventable.

Every life saved from the grip of infectious disease was now seen as simply what Western culture believed it was owed, or at least what we expected as our baseline of normalcy. We were no longer shocked and grateful for such recoveries; rather, we expected them. And similarly, death was no longer an accepted fact of . . . well, life. Now it was reconfigured as a tragic loss that somebody, somewhere, somehow could have or should have prevented. I'll say more about the shift to seeing death as defeat rather than an inevitability in a minute, but for now I want to focus on that dangling carrot of health that germ theory held in front of us.

Of course, I don't mean to deny that on an individual level people still mourned losses in their families and communities before understanding of germ theory abounded. What I'm speaking about here are broad cultural understandings of illness, health, and death as gains or losses—as givens or near misses—and I'm convinced Western society as a whole began to drastically change their attitudes about these things at this time, both from what I know of germ theory's history and from what cognitive psychology can tell us about human nature generally.

The sheer number of products advertised in this period proclaiming to kill germs fully and completely clearly marks this shift. The next chapter is entirely devoted to discussing these products and their aims, but for now, by the 1880s, magazine margins practically burst with goods proclaiming their ability to cleanse all bacteria from anything and everything. Remember the "sanitation theater" I mentioned in chapter 2? This is where it begins. But here's the problem:

LESSON 13:
It ain't whack-a-mole.

In many ways, this builds on **Lesson 6 (Risk elimination is impossible)**. I firmly believe that when society developed germ theory, we gave ourselves the blessing of the foundations of modern medicines (shout-out to antibiotics—hey girl!) and simultaneously the curse of deeply believing that risk elimination *is* possible. After all, if we kill all the germs, we can't get sick, right? The logic is technically sound, but achieving this is realistically impossible. I've started calling this the "whack-a-mole" fallacy: the idea that because something is technically possible, it is also therefore physically achievable. You can keep whacking those suckers, but the very nature of the game guarantees that they'll just keep coming. So, yes, I suppose that if we could rid ourselves of every germ in existence, humans would no longer suffer from infectious disease, but this is simply not possible. The pursuit of this goal at its most extreme can lead to cases of obsessive-compulsive disorder with classic fears of contamination and compulsive hand-washing. Taking this fact to its logical conclusion is maddening. There are some truths that simply have to remain theoretical.

Unsurprisingly, one thing I've heard during the COVID-19 pandemic is that many people who suffer from an obsessive-compulsive disorder that causes them to fear contamination are struggling more than ever. They look around, and it has suddenly become harder and harder to believe that their ceaseless battle against germs is irrational. This has been one of the psychological impacts (remember **Lesson 6**? We contain multitudes, and "risk elimination" is simply a choice of which risks we encounter) I've witnessed during the pandemic, and it comes from the whack-a-mole bias that sends us out of control on the futile path of risk elimination. Interestingly, I've also heard that people with OCD feel more understood than ever (a small victory for those of us working to destigmatize mental health issues), as more and more people have suddenly jumped aboard the impossible Germ Destruction Train bound for Psychic Doomsville. Do not pass Go, do not collect $200. Because, of course, we simply cannot sanitize everything perfectly. There will always be one particle left somewhere, and all it takes is for that particle to touch a finger, and the finger to touch a nose, and the nose to brush a Kleenex that wafts by someone's ankle (recall the deadly linens from our cholera chapter). Complete germ elimination is simply an impossible task, like counting the stars of the sky (by the way, the Victorians tried that, too, so let's not allow their futile tasks to become our own).

Which brings us to

LESSON 14:
Ironically, the "medical revolution" has caused us to live in denial of death.

Bear with me here. The next point is going to seem contradictory. Just keep calm and remember prospect theory. It's important to point out that the widespread faith in germ theory was only possible because society in the 1880s had begun, decades earlier, to see science as the new guiding belief system in an increasingly secularized society. I'm not making any claims here about whether that secularization was good or bad—I'm simply saying that in my experience studying cultural history, people never simply let go of religion, they rather find new things to guide their behaviors and actions; essentially, they create new religions out of secular things. In the late 1800s, this new guiding force was science, and faith in science as a means of solving all the world's most complex problems (even today we call the study of government political *science*, so you can see that this mindset still pervades our society) allowed people to indulge in the fantasy of germ whack-a-mole.

And, of course, handwashing and antiseptic techniques *do* reduce contagious disease transmission, so fortunately and unfortunately (yes, I mean both at once), the fallacy of playing whack-a-mole with germs reaped positive rewards to some extent, but also allowed society to take the delusion of a germ-free life too far. This sort of thinking is a logical fallacy called an "appeal to ignorance."[6] An appeal to ignorance occurs when we have been doing something to ward off a negative effect, and when said negative effect never happens, we are all too easily able to assume (possibly incorrectly) that our actions *prevented* the unwanted event from occurring. For instance, say you light a candle every night to prevent a catastrophic hurricane from occurring in Indiana. The fact that you do this every night, and a hurricane has never struck Indiana, would enable a fervent believer in the candle's powers to say it was the candle-lighting ritual that prevented the hurricane. A similar form of magical thinking pervaded society in the 1880s, when sanitation theater seemed more likely than ever to have a real effect on life. You'll recall that sanitary methods existed prior to germ theory, but antiseptic chemicals could be more effectively developed at this point. Additionally, people were simply more inclined to believe that their overuse was helpful. Doing so *did* decrease infectious disease rates—but it could never eliminate them fully, and therein lies the problem.

Based on my research, I believe that the broad cultural knowledge that disease rates *had* dropped is precisely what allowed this risk elimi-

---

6   This is a common philosophical concept. A concise definition can be found on Texas State University's Philosophy Department webpage on Appeals and Informal Fallacies, www.txstate.edu/philosophy/resources/fallacy-definitions/Appeal -to-Ignorance.html.

nation bias to spin out of control and keep society thinking that if a little sanitation had helped keep people healthy, then more was necessarily both possible and better—that there could never be too much sanitation, in fact. A century and a half later, we are now a society that has sanitized death itself, metaphorically speaking. As the West saw fewer and fewer deaths from infectious disease, this reinforced the idea that our whack-a-mole game was working, leading us to be even *more* risk averse and to double down on our risk-elimination practices because of the appeal to ignorance fallacy. It's a perpetual motion machine; the less familiar with death we become in society, largely because of germ theory–based antiseptic practices, the more we mistake such risk mitigation practices for the feasibility of total risk *elimination*. This seems to be working, because when we see less death around us, we grow more fearful of death as a concept and less willing to accept it as a given fact of all biological life. In short, we have become not only obsessed with risk elimination but totally risk *averse*. Our privileged safety from disease has ironically weakened us by making us much too fearful of death. It's a deadly strategy that allows us the fantasy of feeling safe, but only if we maintain a state of constant hypervigilance (recall **Lesson 6** and you'll remember that this is unsustainable and self-defeating).

Even in the 1880s, society used to have a healthy host of rituals surrounding death that we've all but lost in our desire to pretend it doesn't exist. We've robbed ourselves even of the psychic means of coping with death, so deeply do we want to pretend it won't come for us. Death is something unfamiliar to us—we don't see it every day like Montagu, Defoe, Snow, and Semmelweis did—and so it becomes the preeminent goal of daily life to avoid death at all costs. There's that whack-a-mole game again. Sooner or later, we all die. And if we lived in a society more capable of accepting that, we could probably find a comfortable middle zone where we could also accept that, as one *At-*

lantic article noted in May 2020, "an all-or-nothing approach to risk prevention" is failing.[7] If we could embrace this fact, we might be able to see that

LESSON 15:
Life is like a box of chocolates—er, a garden.

We *need* bacteria! Our risk elimination compulsion is psychologically and existentially dangerous. But, beyond this, if we take the lessons of chapter 3 to heart, there are dire physical consequences to treating microbes like a whack-a-mole game. As I've mentioned earlier, the goal of One Health is to demonstrate that all humans' fates are interconnected, and that animal health is interconnected with that of humans. To that, people are beginning to add microbial health as interconnected with that of humans. I work regularly with a team of researchers and educators from across the United States as a part of the iAMResponsible Project who are working to combat antimicrobial resistance using a One Health model: raising public awareness about the interconnectedness of humans, animals, microbes, and the environment so that we will all be able to work together to protect the efficacy of antibiotics for future generations. Of course, viruses and bacteria aren't the same thing, and antibiotics are ineffective against viruses. However, since viral and bacterial pathogens are often discussed together, and because the history of bacteriology is older, giving us more historical examples to work with, it makes sense to draw from our understandings of bacteria as a means to contemplate bacterial *and* viral

---

7   Julia Marcus, "Quarantine Fatigue Is Real," *Atlantic*, May 11, 2020, www.the atlantic.com/ideas/archive/2020/05/quarantine-fatigue-real-and-shaming-people -wont-help/611482/.

threats to humanity. Through my work with this team, I've had the somewhat horrifying privilege of learning just how much humanity's growing obsession with sanitation theater is dooming us. Now, with regard to the novel coronavirus, there are some very obvious efficacy problems with such sanitation theater, particularly because the virus is only rarely transmitted via contaminated surfaces. But even more generally, we have a great deal of evidence that even sanitizing surfaces in hospitals—where germ-free surfaces are obviously important—is slowly inching us toward the robot apocalypse. Just kidding, I mean the antibiotic resistance apocalypse. (Sorry, but I figured I should lighten the mood a bit because it's about to get dark.)

Antibiotics do occur naturally, in soils and such, which is how we were able to discover and harness them for human purposes. But just like anything, bacteria evolve, and the more we use antibiotics, the more frequently a select few bacteria will achieve immunity to antibiotic drugs. Those bacteria then have babies (well, technically they undergo binary fission, but you get the idea), and pretty soon there are more and more bacteria that go Hulk on our antibiotics. Cue rampant human death. Increasingly, scientists are discovering that even just the use of cleansing products—like hand sanitizers and bleach—put pressure on the minute ecosystems in which bacteria live, inadvertently killing only those bacteria that can't evolve defenses and leaving a race of superbacteria against which we will one day find our current medicines useless. I hope that this far into this book, you're beginning to realize just how terrifying that would be, because lemme tell you, bacteria are pretty darn scary.

Now, I know what you're thinking: Didn't I just say that risk elimination is impossible and we shouldn't live in such fear of bacteria that we go into whack-a-mole mode? That's true. But it's also true that releasing our vise grip on risk aversion *just enough* that we can lay down the whack-a-mole hammer might be the key to our very survival as a species. We know that antibiotic overuse kills good healthy bacteria that the body needs, for instance. In fact, overuse of some antibiotics kills enough good gut bacteria that it can cause *C. difficile* infections—an awful GI bug that results from the elimination of good bacteria that would naturally be culling overpopulations of bad bacteria (similar to how predatory animals like wolves naturally prevent overpopulation of animals like deer that can strip forestland bare). Obviously, more antibiotics won't solve problems like *C. difficile*—in fact, one of the most revolutionary treatments has been something called fecal transplants, which is exactly what it sounds like. Good bacteria that live in excrement are harvested, put into pills, and swallowed, allowing good bacteria to reign supreme once more in the besieged gut. Studies on hospital surfaces have similarly found that purposefully colonizing hospital surfaces with *good* bacteria can eliminate disease-causing germs just as effectively as sanitizing chemicals, without the unwanted side effect of increasing antibiotic resistance. Several notable scholars in the field have called this "Bidirectional Hygiene," or "Bygiene." This essentially consists of the introduction of beneficial species in the environment that are able to counteract the colonization from pathogenic microorganisms.[8] Bacteria can be cultivated like gardens, and if we could take our anxious fingers off the kill switch for a moment, we could weed our gardens carefully instead of frantically employing a slash-and-burn approach.

Bacteria—like our mindsets—live in a careful balance where extremes of any kind set things off kilter and spinning out of control. I've said this repeatedly so far about political extremes, and about seeing those who disagree with us as archetypal villains. The same is also true about our personal and existential beliefs: finding the middle

---

8   Maria D'Accolti, Irene Soffritti, Sante Mazzacane, and Elisabetta Caselli, "Fighting AMR in the Healthcare Environment: Microbiome-Based Sanitation Approaches and Monitoring Tools," *International Journal of Molecular Science* 20 (2019).

zone is key. At Whitworth University, where I currently teach, we call this path of moderation "the narrow ridge," and I think the metaphor is apt.[9] We have to find a middle road between escalating our germ elimination efforts too much and the obviously undesirable extreme of feeling helpless in the face of bacteria. Eventually, the Victorians themselves learned that bacterial cultivation was vital to properly controlling disease-causing sewage. When the right bacteria were allowed to thrive, they helped naturally break down waste that otherwise wreaked havoc on society. Now in 2021, we need to find that middle road again, because bacteria, too, live in a careful balance of helpful and harmful organisms, and we humans, as a species, also live in a careful balance with these bacteria. Gardens also take time to grow. In the hospital study mentioned above, spores took months to repopulate enough to control bacteria. Alas, here another element of popular culture unfortunately has contributed to these problems, namely our need for instant gratification. Careful stewardship of the macro- and microscopic gardens in which we all dwell will require looking toward the future and initiating proactive programs like this that may not deliver an immediate payoff but will ultimately heal us physically and psychically. It would require letting go of the whack-a-mole desires that cause us to long for quick and complete results, which have brought with them even more baggage, as I'll address in the next chapter.

BUT FIRST . . .

---

9 Beck Taylor, "Whitworth's Enduring Commitments to Mind and Heart," inaugural address, October 10, 2020, www.whitworth.edu/cms/administration/president-beck-a-taylor/speeches-and-messages/inaugural-address/.

INTERLUDE

THE ANTI-CHAPTER

══

LET'S TALK ABOUT DEATH, BABY

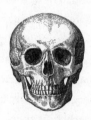

Let's talk about you and me,
Let's talk about all the good things
and the bad things that may be,
Let's talk about death.

Yes, I have been known to open class with this personally improvised rendition of the 1991 Salt-N-Pepa classic. No, I didn't ask for your opinion about that particular teaching strategy.

Actually, I have asked for it, by writing and publishing this book and circulating this knowledge in the world. That's been the hardest part of writing this entire book—not writing it itself. I have no problem banging out a set number of words per day under a tight deadline. It's my weird, and possibly very boring, X-Men power. Anyway, the writing isn't hard, but saying what I think may be unpopular is. Like most humans, I really want people to like me, probably too much so. But desperate times call for desperate measures, and it's time to put my money where my mouth has been, so to speak, and own up to my opinions about death.

Yes, I sometimes make light of it with shenanigans like the one above. I even regularly wear death-themed jewelry, ranging from authentic Victorian mourning earrings to modern-day skeleton-shaped hair clips and rings shaped like coffins. And I don't think this makes me irreverent. I want death to be something we talk about *more*. I want all of us to reflect on its mystery, and what it can teach us about living the life we want now, here, today. I want Americans to talk about it so much that it's not taboo. In the present moment, I've worn my coffin ring and skeleton barrette a lot less, for fear of offending anyone who has either recently lost someone or, more to the point for me (since death has always existed for people, inside and outside of pandemics), who might be living in constant fear of losing someone in the 2020 pandemic. I worry that this jewelry might trigger panic and fear in the present societal moment. But such jewelry and icons were once quite common. They're called *memento mori* and were meant to remind anyone who saw them of the impermanence of life. At times, there was almost certainly a religious element to the *memento*, warning pious Christians to look to the afterlife and prepare themselves on earth for the life after death.

But it's also a really effective reminder, religious or not, that we all come to the same end. It keeps me mindful of my actions here and now, and it's also a personal cognitive-behavioral mechanism I introduced into my own life to get rid of my own fears of death, which at various times in my life have completely debilitated me. That lengthy story is for another book, but I mention it briefly here as a form of my credentials: I'm not just one of those magical people who don't fear their own death. You know the people. We hear about these folks, and even encounter them sometimes—people who can bravely acknowledge that we all die, and who seem to not ever really worry about it. I'm not that. Honestly, I don't know if I'll ever fully understand how to completely experience that sort of bravery, but I do know that we ought to try.

So, yes, I have lived years—years!—of my life in the shadow of a stultifying fear of death, and perhaps more than my time spent studying death and disease, this is my most compelling qualification that enables me to tell you this: We have to stop fearing death. Living in a constant fear of death is no kind of life. I've said as much briefly in **Lessons 6 and 14**, but it's an important enough point about where our path *out* of pandemic lies that it's worth devoting an entire anti-chapter to. You read that right: accepting our mortality could very well be the most important factor in leading us away from the death on a massive scale that we're witnessing during the COVID-19 pandemic.

Our lifestyle in the Western world, in which we're privileged to not see much death around us, has ironically led to an existence where we cannot tolerate the idea of death. As I've written in *YES!* magazine, living in denial of death will backfire, every time. Why? Because we will all die.

Death and taxes (and disease), remember?

For pretty much the first time in human history, life since the 1950s has been relatively free of death, and certainly free of very many epidemics of infectious disease, at least in the developed world. As I've explained in the past few chapters, this allows us to problematically pretend that death simply won't come for us. In America, even as compared to our other Western European counterparts, we use hospice services far too infrequently, and far too readily attempt to extend life forever, at all costs—particularly at the cost of the quality of our emotional, psychological, and social life. Many popular authors are beginning to discuss cultivating a new culture of death in America, most notably Caitlin Doughty in *Smoke Gets in Your Eyes*, who points out that we have invented the entire funerary industry to avoid facing the realities of death. As I said in my previously mentioned magazine article, we want to "cart away death"—to get it out of our faces, away from our homes, and, with modern-day embalming and cosmetics, to make the dead appear living again for our last viewing of them.[1] It may be a bit extreme to say that the entire funeral industry arose for this purpose, because it was growing even in the Victorian era, when death was readily confronted. In fact, the Victorian funerary industry was in many ways a business designed to create a *spectacle* of death, rather than to hide it, and included dramatic rituals such as hiring random people to be mourners in a loved one's funeral procession. Nevertheless, I agree with Doughty, yet I think it's more than accurate to say that

---

1 Kari Nixon, "Why I Wore Black After He Died," *YES!*, October 2, 2019, www.yesmagazine.org/issue/death/opinion/2019/10/02/grief-dying -mourning-victorian-culture/.

the funeral industry has *become* an industry devoted to hiding death. Indeed, in carting away death, I would argue that our sanitation theater has caused us to "scrub . . . society clean of anything that bespeaks death. . . . Yet by privileging ourselves with this social sanitation that offers a fantasy of life free from death, we have, in fact, robbed ourselves of any means of coping with it."[2]

That is, in pragmatically relieving ourselves of the burden of dealing with death, we have, I think, also robbed ourselves of the rituals that humans use to cope with loss emotionally. Victorians made a spectacle of mourning and death by constructing an entire industry around it. When teaching, I compare it to the size of the modern-day marriage industry, as both could be equally excessively extravagant. There was mourning stationery, with black borders that told letter recipients that their correspondent had encountered a loss, even if the letter content itself had nothing to do with the subject. There were mourning fabrics to put on carriages, not to mention, of course, the black clothes and jewelry women wore (men wore black armbands). Families kept the body of their departed in their home for at least a week, and clocks were stopped for the same period. I think these rituals are beautiful—they demonstrate concretely that a family's rhythms have been stopped (the clocks) and are having to rebuild themselves (the stationery, the carriage décor) around an absence, like a tree regrafting itself together after a lightning strike splits it at its core. There were rituals of final connection with the departed, too. Families washed the bodies themselves, spending a final mo-

---

2   Ibid.

ment with their departed, and they sometimes took one last picture of the body.

Imagine our world if a simple black flag on your car or a black, weighted line at the end of your e-mail signature silently signaled to the world, *I am grieving. My world has altered forever. I cannot speak my pain, but it is eating me alive. I am not whole. I may never be whole again.* How different things might look! To have your pain known in your support network without having to utter the unutterable sinkhole of grief that's sucking you into its abyss—to me, that sounds like about the only soothing balm that might begin to comfort the heart adrift in the torrents of death.

Having something physical to mark my loss has also helped me through moments when death brushed against my life, leaving ragged emotional bruises in every spot it touched. For me, the most mysterious—the most horrible—part of death is that the *everything* of loss is marked only by *nothingness*—a "human-shaped hole in the universe."[3] The world ticks on, but your own private world has stopped in its tracks, and there is nothing to mark the weighty absence of the person who should still be filling your life. Victorians also used to clip a lock of hair from the departed to make into jewelry for themselves, to remember their loved one by. My students usually find this disgusting, and I have to admit that the levels of intricacy with which Victorians would weave corpse-hair into art can be a little . . . shocking. But I've done

3   Kari Nixon, "Grieving Our Collective Loss, One Stitch at a Time," *YES!*, May 1, 2020, www.yesmagazine.org/opinion/2020/05/01/coronavirus -death-grief/.

it myself when my dog died. As I said in my article devoted to his death, "I too clipped a lock of his hair and stored it away in an envelope to be sent to the few people who still practice the art of weaving Victorian hair jewelry for mourners. It's not off-putting to me, because it was him—a cherished life connected to mine. It's the last remaining vestige of his DNA—why wouldn't I hoard it greedily when I've been deprived of every other part of his presence?"[4]

The emptiness, the abstract gone-ness of someone who was such a presence in our lives is the worst part of death, if you ask me. During the early months of the COVID-19 pandemic, I knitted a blanket, using a stitch for every ten deaths globally, simply so I could hold something in my hands that could allow me to feel *some actual weight of loss*.[5]

Forgive me for returning to my favorite hair clip. It was made by a local artist, Summer Hightower, at the Veda Lux boutique here in Spokane, Washington (it doesn't feel right not to plug her, since she hand-makes all her own jewelry, and she's a true artist). The clip is a heather-gray Victorian-style brooch, with a skeleton hand clutching it. I'm absolutely enamored with it, because it sums up everything I wish I could communicate here, thoughts that I passionately believe would help us look at disease and, yes, even the current pandemic differently, and possibly not only survive it but also survive it in better shape. That hair clip represents so much: the beautiful and the broken melded together. Isn't that what we all are, at some level? Beautiful and flawed—it sums up every unique

4 Nixon, "Why I Wore Black."

5 Nixon, "Grieving Our Collective Loss."

life that ever was on this planet. It sums up life itself. It sums up death itself, for death is only mourned because of a beautiful, "never-to-be-had-again" life lost.[6] We are all beautifully flawed. So is life. And so is death, because it is a part of life, and vice versa. The two seemingly opposed halves merge into a holistic entity so that one cannot be taken without the other.

No one could argue that this means *seeking* death; rather it entails simply accepting death as it is: a fact of life. Having life means eventually having to die. We've problematically separated the two in our imaginations—not consciously, of course, but by the practices that define our society and impact our subconscious thinking. Western society got into tricky territory because once we separated them out, defining them as two discrete states rather than an interconnected state of being, we then applied value judgments to them. We began to falsely align our natural grief responses to death with the problematic fallacy of seeing death as a failure of society rather than a given fact of every existence ever.

Of course, we can and should mourn death—each and every death that has ever happened in the history of humanity represents the loss of a unique life that will never be captured again. The rhythmic fading away of human life over the course of history reminds me of the feeling I get when I watch my daughters blow soap bubbles in the summer evenings. Watching every bubble, each ephemerally beautiful and tragically unique in its own way, float away or burst represents a moment that can never be reclaimed. But mourning a life can still be done *mindfully*, with the awareness before, during, and

---

6 Ibid.

after, that death is the most natural thing of all, second only to being born, although we have shorn it of all the rituals that ought to mark this momentous transition, just as we mark other birth and growth milestones.

Like I've said, there are plenty of people making moves in this direction, but one way I incorporate this into my own life is using my *memento mori* as a form of rational emotive behavior therapy. In REBT, a form of cognitive behavioral therapy (CBT), patients are taught to identify subtly occurring automatic, all-or-nothing thoughts, such as "I have to make an A on this test or I'm never going to get into medical school." Once a person can identify that they are subconsciously allowing such automatic thoughts to color their perspectives, they then learn to stop the thought and consciously think differently.[7] For instance, one could reframe the previous thought as: "I have no idea if this test will really prevent all my career goals, and it's unlikely that one test alone could have such a large impact upon my life." Although REBT was adopted as a psychological practice before mindfulness and meditation were very well studied, I find the two schools of thought related; mindfulness suggests that allowing ourselves to observe our own thoughts rationally and without emotion can help us cope. Remember the pendulum swing of denial and panic I mentioned in **Lesson 6**? Mindfulness takes the middle road, as it were, as its weapon of choice to counter the problematic impact of such extreme thoughts (it does a lot of other things, too, of course). REBT, for its part, acknowledges that the little ways we think about our world and our lives impact the way

---

7   Jordan Harp, personal communication.

we behave, and these behaviors then cycle back to impact the way we feel about things, and so on. So, from my perspective, a subtle denial of death in our culture—where we simply don't see it or talk about it much—absolutely facilitates our implicit cultural feelings that death is the ultimate defeat, to be avoided at all costs.

Having a piece of Victorian mourning jewelry on me is my "checkpoint" for unemotionally identifying the fact that I'm going through my day with the automatic denial of my own and my loved ones' mortality, and for correcting this automatic thought with the conscious, mindful awareness that we will all die. My favorite philosopher to teach my students is Julia Kristeva, whose concept of "abjection" I find very useful in explaining the impact of this practice from a more existential perspective (should you for some reason dislike CBT and mindfulness approaches). I'll spare you the confusing 1980s French philosophy lingo—which I have it on authority from a French therapist of mine is just as confusing in the original French—and give you the TL;DR version. Kristeva says that we live in constant denial of things that we associate with "not us" (these things she terms "the abject"). I teach it to my students like this: think of what you were like in high school. If you were anything like me, you saw yourself in fairly cut-and-dried terms. I was smart, so I saw myself as, by definition, not sporty. I was preppy, therefore I was not goth, and so forth. These things that seemed by definition opposed to who I was (or saw myself as) were my "abject." For Kristeva, the ultimate "abject," which we spend our entire lives believing is completely opposed to our own identity, is anything that signifies our capacity to die. Of course, we do this so that we aren't frozen in fear, wondering if every stop sign or school campus holds a fatal accident or mass shooting.

But Kristeva's point—or at least what I make of it in my teaching—is that if we could blend the "I/not I" together and accept them as a unified whole, we wouldn't be frozen in fear to begin with. For instance, if I had had a less limiting view of myself in high school (as a smart person who could not, by virtue of this fact, possibly be interested in sports), I might have discovered that I loved sports. I might have become a very different person than the overly sedentary scholar that I am today, with creaky hips at thirty-four. To use a different example, if we could all embrace that we all have a *little* emo inside of us, and probably some preppy, too, then we wouldn't have to have such divisive categories defining our styles and boxing them in with external ideas of what "goth" is and is not.

For Kristeva, all of this can be applied to our deep desire to believe we won't die . . . at least not anytime soon (another version of the same denial). For Kristeva, if we could see life as a continuum of states rather than a binary of living/dead, we could live more holistically: we'd be, existentially speaking, the sporty nerd or the gothic-prep, the yin to our own yang. We could hold our mortality neatly in tension with our current life, without distress. Instead, we tend to try to react to our capacity to die with denial, which only fuels our fear. All of this, by the way, is simply another way of describing the beautiful/broken dynamic I mentioned earlier, but it's a tricky point, which is why I'm repeating it a few different ways. I find my students need several repetitions of the idea to accept it, because it's frankly just hard to overcome decades of a social fantasy that trains us to believe that denying the reality of our own mortality is a useful means of coping with our fear of that mortality. For Kristeva, and according to CBT, REBT, and mindfulness therapies, we are far, far better off accepting our mortality fully.

What does this have to do with COVID-19, or any future epidemics for that matter? Well, first of all, this is the anti-chapter, which means I get to do what I want without fear of defending its relevance. Just kidding. It has a lot to do with COVID-19, but in ways that aren't tied to any specific epidemic and have more to do with what our society believes about human life and death in the wake of the germ theory revolution of the 1880s.

I mentioned this before in **Lesson 6**, but it's worth saying again here, and with different words. We are not solely biological beings. We are bio-psycho-socio-emotional beings. There are certain things in life—like death—that are just going to be terrible. Like death itself, the ripping, clawing teeth of grief are another almost guarantee, if we've been blessed to have anyone we've loved in our lives, pets included. In these times of emotional pain and social loss, what do we have besides our social network to support us?

During my undergraduate days, I did a research paper on the Book of Job, which is honestly a super-depressing Bible book in which a guy's life falls apart around him—he loses absolutely everything. Truly, everything. His livestock are stolen. His kids die. And then, adding insult to injury, he gets covered with boils. Why I picked that particular text to write a paper on as a college student I'm not sure, except to say that I guess I was always fascinated with the darker elements that necessarily cling to all the light of existence. My favorite part of Job at the time was in chapter 2, when Job is covered with boils (I guess I've always liked disease, too), and his friends come and sit with him. They don't talk. They don't do anything. They're just with him. They see that the enormity of his grief and the weight of the tragedy that has befallen him can't actually be fixed by anything they do. But they're there. Because in the wake of unavoidable physical illness or death, what else do we have but the people who are still in our circle?[8]

Ironically, though, when we live a life in denial of death, we live a life that focuses only on death entirely—as Kristeva says, everything becomes defined by the "not I" that we're trying to hide from to begin with. In this state, then, we begin to try to uphold a fantasy of a purely biological life through our attempts to preserve this (and only this) part of human life. When we do this, we deny our very selves the value we could be placing on the social and emotional aspects of our world. Without even communal rituals to see us through or to concretize our grief, we deny ourselves the comforts of friendship and community because we've lived a life focused on denying their necessity and have instead aimed only at preserving a beating heart and pumping lungs. Yet since death will strike all of our lives at some point, we've only set ourselves up for failure. We can't avoid death, and in trying to do so, we've only succeeded at avoiding one another. We *need* one another. We are social creatures (**Lesson 12**), and to live within a fantasy of a death-free life will ultimately reduce our lives to the biological elements we've imagined them to be. We become

---

8 To be fair, his friends are pretty crummy pals in a lot of ways. I still love this moment, though.

mere lumps of flesh that will still inevitably die, that have cut themselves off from the comforts of community, friendship, and family.

During the pandemic, I've become accustomed to saying that humans are my most and least favorite part of humanity. Italians singing to one another from balconies during quarantine, artists playing concerts on YouTube, celebrities reading bedtime stories for children. We're capable of such beauty. We're also capable of such atrocities—I need not outline them here, in a chapter already addressing the very dark matter of death. Sometimes we muddle it up in less obviously horrific ways, though. I get why we try not to think about our own deaths, or the deaths of those we love most. It's terrifying, and I've personally lived parts of my life alternating between trying to run from this terror or being frozen in place by it. It's something of a knee-jerk reaction for most living beings, I'd say, to varying degrees. And yet that very protective instinct to deny what frightens us, in the case of pandemic disease in 2020 and death more generally, has set us up for failure. For if we could fold death flexibly into our concept of life, we could so much more easily feel out the "middle path" that we need to walk along today (more on this coming up in **Lesson 18**). Somewhere between totally denying that COVID-19 exists and refusing all contact until a vaccine is created, there's a middle zone that's sustainable. This middle zone, should we choose to seek it out, might very well be capable of tolerating risk along with the understanding that humans need humans. It might be able to acknowledge that choosing social and emotional distress for the preservation of biological life is indeed a cost-benefit analysis. I hardly proclaim to know what this middle ground looks like. Instead, I believe in the beauty of human ingenuity and creativity to be able to find it when many of us approach the same problem. But I believe we can do so only when we move outside the centrifugal force of denial-panic and find a stable approach that accepts death not as a failure but as evidence of wondrous life.

AND NOW BACK TO . . .

6

DESPERATE REMEDIES AND DANGEROUS CURES THROUGHOUT HISTORY

*How Risk Aversion Paradoxically
Leads to Risky Behaviors*

═══

1875-1901

Mrs. J hunched over, lightly clutching her stomach with her right hand, adopting what was increasingly becoming her standard posture. Her abdominal pain was right next to her in the surgical waiting room, like a trusty sidekick, she thought. No, she corrected her own imaginings, it was more like a haunting specter. She seemed more wedded to the pain than to her husband, so loyally devoted was—well, whatever was causing the pain. Dr. H assured her, however, that the pain would stop soon, once he removed her gallbladder. Although she believed him, she did wonder at the hissing sound she heard coming from some equipment in the surgery room. What could that be about?

═══

Now, if this were a movie, this is the moment where the all-seeing eye of the camera would pan into the next room and show the viewer the contraption Mrs. J had heard, rigged up to spray acid into her viscera while she was prone on the operating table.

Of course, Mrs. J never existed. I've adopted here the Victorian practice of using initials to signal imaginary case studies. Her story is representative of a set of cultural shifts that occurred as germ theory and antiseptics became more widespread in society. What we can learn from the imaginary Mrs. J, the doctors that would have served her, and the whole host of patients that would have been seeking medical advice and solutions at this time are that

Lesson 16:   Panaceas are predictable.

Lesson 17:   Science is not a saint.

Lesson 18:   There is no "real" world except what we make.

After the invention of anesthesia, elective surgeries became more and more common. The playwright George Bernard Shaw (whose play *Pygmalion* is the basis for the musical *My Fair Lady*, and who always has a place in my heart because of his special brand of beautiful snark) particularly insisted that the development of anesthesia itself enabled doctors to market surgeries like never before. Because people could be put under, he argued, they were more willing to undergo elective surgeries than before general anesthetic techniques existed. His logic makes sense. The idea of being awake and *feeling* someone cut into your body would likely make most of us avoid surgery unless it was absolutely necessary, and maybe even still then.

Still, the use of generalized anesthesia came with its own bundle of concerns. Patients worried and fretted about what doctors might do to unconscious bodies during surgery. Stories of rape and other forms of assault abounded in newspapers. What possibly few of these patients knew, though, and even fewer of them would have even objected to regardless, was that corrosive acid would be sprayed into their bodies during the entirety of their surgical procedures, to protect against contamination. Special devices were invented just for the purpose of gently misting carbolic acid (the nineteenth-century version of bleach) throughout an operating room, the goal being that the chemical could purify both the surgeons' lungs and the patients' insides at the same time.[1]

Like anesthesia's insidious ability to make elective, non-lifesaving surgeries more widely marketable, the allure of quick fixes through pills and cure-alls seems to be fairly universal. In particular, during the course of my research, I've noticed a decided uptick in the marketing of medical panaceas (that's a fancy word for "this will cure everything") in the mid-1800s. Some of this is likely due to the fact that magazines themselves—the main form in which product advertisements appeared—were becoming more common around that time. It was simply easier to advertise products to begin with. But I also suspect that a big reason medical cure-alls were a booming business during that period is because germ theory provided an easy scientific framework to justify or explain curatives in a way that seemed reasonable to a society desperate for answers (like spraying acid into bodily cavities to supposedly make surgery safer).

The brazen confidence of germ theory introduced a host of outrageous products claiming to be the solution to germs. People seemed to suddenly think, *Aha! Germ theory has shown us that disease-causing organisms are alive? Great! All we have to do is kill them and we'll have it made!* (See **Lesson 13**). Cue hundreds of products meant to help

---

1   In fact, the Material Safety Data Sheet for carbolic acid describes it as "toxic . . . if swallowed . . . in contact with skin . . . [or] inhaled," and notes that it "may cause damage to organs through prolonged or repeated exposure . . . [especially to the] kidney, liver, skin, [and] nervous system," essentially warning modern users to be extremely careful with the substance. It's astounding to think that Victorians did *all of these things* regularly and on purpose.

people inhale, ingest, or inject antiseptics into their bodies. I've already mentioned one of Victorians' favorite tools: carbolic acid. Victorians invented endless methods of trying to inhale it or diffuse it into a room. The Carbolic Smoke Ball was a very popular product—a solid ball of the stuff that could be lit, like incense, and either inhaled directly into the nose or left to diffuse and cleanse a home.

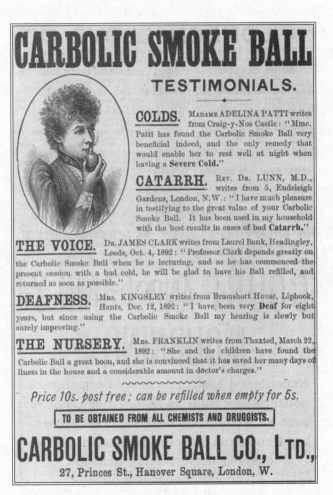

"Carbolic Smoke Ball," *Sketch* 4 (1893), p. 108.

There are many more products of this nature, meant to cleanse every inch of human bodies and the natural environment of contaminating germs. I personally own a product that was manufactured during this period that looks something like a small kerosene lamp. The owner was instructed to put antiseptic chemicals into the basin above the flame, as a sort of antiseptic diffuser meant to purify the germs from the air in the house. (I'll take essential oils over boiled, diffused acid any day, thankyouverymuch.) For those who preferred ingested purification, "blood purifying" pills were absolutely everywhere, persuading consumers that each and every cell of blood could and needed to be cleansed of germs. There were antimicrobial hand towels for cleaning, antiseptic paints for cleansing or preventing disease, and even raincoats touted as having antibacterial properties. The desire for and advertised possibility of perfectly sanitizing one's environment was seemingly endless.

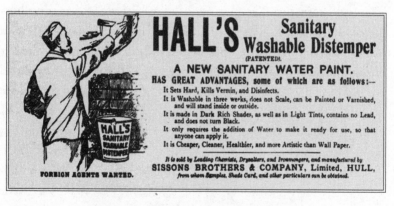

"Hall's Sanitary Washable Distemper: A New Sanitary
Water Paint," *Strand Magazine* 18 (1899), p. xxxix.

In most of my years of teaching, my students have seen such products as ridiculous. However, as the novel coronavirus is now demonstrating, and as I have long tried to show my students, this is only a logical outcome of a society that (1) understands only a few basic facts about the pathogens that are killing them, but (2) is confident that somehow, some way, they can vanquish their foes.

One of the reasons I love teaching the Victorians as a means to understanding our own world is that they simultaneously provide examples of behaviors that, to us, seem easily recognizable as ridiculous, extreme, or misguided, while also providing a useful case study by which to reframe or reconsider our own practices. It's quite easy to scoff at something someone did 150 years ago and assume that we'd never fall prey to equally silly ideas. But are the ideas behind many of our alternative therapies any different? If anything existed that truly cured everything, we wouldn't still be searching around for the next cure-all, and there wouldn't be any more disease.

Once more, for the people in the back: there will always be disease.

And alternative therapies aren't the only thing we see contributing to the whack-a-mole fallacy today. Products proclaiming, with Victorian-style confidence, an ability to fully cleanse germs—whether in the air, on our counters, or in our bodies—are still everywhere. We *still* have hand towels touting strands of antimicrobial silver. I see plastic products all the time with packaging promoting antimicrobial coatings that prevent germ contamination. Different vitamins and supplements routinely claim to be able to "detoxify" the body, which is not so very different from the "blood purifying" pills of yore. So can we honestly say we've moved beyond the "silly" Victorian panaceas of the past?

No such tool exists that will fully cleanse our bodies or our world of germs. But, as we've seen already, it's human nature to take the limited information we have in a life-or-death situation (antiseptic methods kill coronavirus) and sometimes apply it too extensively and inappropriately (drinking bleach). This chapter's first lesson is simply that

LESSON 16:
Panaceas are predictable.

When we look at the past—especially if we look to our Victorian fore-bears, who were the first people to live with the knowledge that we exist perpetually in a sea of germs—we can see that such extreme responses are in fact rather predictable outcomes of desperate people. In this light, these responses might not seem so extreme after all. Rather, they are simply overly extended logical outcomes of the sort of ideas that contaminate modern thinking (**Lesson 13**). I understood (but was also troubled by) the temptation to publicly scoff at the thought of injections of bleach to ward off COVID-19 with silly memes or angry social media posts. Yet if we can dig a little deeper than our desire to post mocking memes, we'll see that the *will*, rather than the *way*, is what we should be focusing on if we want to help our fellow humans through this. Of course, drinking bleach is a horrifyingly dangerous suggestion. But rather than beating our heads against walls about what we perceive as the stupidity of those around us (remember **Lesson 11**?), we'd do more good, I think, if we were to try to explore the *reasons* that such an obviously toxic idea seemed at all reasonable to anyone, anywhere. The irrationality of the suggestion is not the explanation; it should be the question. If something so obviously nonsensical has been brought up at all: Why? What happened to make it seem appealing? Especially to make so many people overlook its obvious inaccuracies?

The answer—as will hardly be news to you if you've been reading this book straight through—is the complex mix of our modern-day scientific framework for understanding disease and the desires for total purity it has ushered into our society. It's the whack-a-mole fallacy at play again; yes, we think subconsciously, drinking poison is dangerous, but so are these germs. And when you throw into that logic a society that has such risk and death aversion that it cannot view life with a garden mentality (**Lessons 14 and 15**), a decent number of people are going to respond to that dilemma by razing the garden entirely. None of this problematic thinking would be possible, however, were it not for a particular set of cultural attitudes about science, which I alluded to in chapter 2. Which brings me to my next point:

LESSON 17:
Science is not a saint.

One of my favorite academic book titles ever is *Never Pure: Historical Studies of Science as If It Was Produced by People with Bodies, Situated in Time, Space, Culture, and Society, and Struggling for Credibility and Authority.* Written by Steven Shapin, this book's title could virtually have been the title of this lesson, were it not for its inconvenient length, which is, of course, Shapin's very point. Just like data, as discussed in **Lesson 6**, science—the discipline that analyzes data—is messy. It is produced by humans who exist in time and space under certain funding and social pressures, all of which produce certain kinds of knowledge that privilege certain viewpoints and are subject to error. What's more, it's all too convenient to abridge this reality into short, digestible sound bites that obscure the fact that science is an inconvenient, tangled mess of data, and it never adheres to our ideas of what would be convenient or simple.

Based on my research into the middle- to late-Victorian period, I believe this is when Enlightenment views of objective knowledge as the gold standard of legitimate science, paired with decreasing religious belief, created the beginnings of our current overvalorization (and misunderstanding) of science. George Levine has argued that in the Victorian period in history, "'scientific knowledge' seemed to be 'beyond prejudice, and claim[ed] the authority lost by religion.'"[2] I heartily agree. When society felt adrift in the wake of its loss of religious belief, people turned to science as the anchor that could stabilize them. Again, this is not an argument about the importance or lack thereof of religion. It's rather a statement that humans seek frameworks by which to guide their understanding of the world, and whether they turn to religion or science or something in between, they'll find *something* to grasp hold of and use to make sense of an often senseless and chaotic world. In my view, we've done that with science over the last 150 years, resulting in many problematic outcomes.

Don't get me wrong—I love science. Remember, I was the girl who thought I could figure out the Path to Paradise using actuarial tables. But we do a great disservice to ourselves and scientists when we don't see science as *Produced by People with Bodies, Situated in Time, Space, Culture, and Society, and Struggling for Credibility and Authority* (that's my new band name). I've personally spoken with many scientists about this, and they fully agree that to see science as some single entity with a capital "S" does not honor the labor they do, day in and day out, at lab benches around the world. You may be saying, "But of course we don't treat science that way—or at least, I don't," but I'm here to tell you that you do. If you've ever shared a "This Week in Science" article on social media, you've fallen victim to this mode of speaking about science. Headlines like "For the First Time, Scientists Detect the Ghostly Signal That Reveals the Engine of the Universe"[3] ignore the tiny bits of data that took years to compile (in this case,

---

2 George Levine, *Realism, Ethics and Secularism: Essays on Victorian Literature and Science* (New Brunswick, NJ: Rutgers University Press, 2009), quoted in Kari Nixon, *Kept from All Contagion*, 110.

3 Tom Metcalfe, "For the First Time, Scientists Detect the Ghostly Signal That Reveals the Engine of the Universe," *NBC Nightly News*, November 25, 2020, www.nbcnews.com/science/space/first-time-scientists-detect-ghostly-signal-reveals-engine-universe-n1248982.

the researchers have been working since 1990). These tiny bits of data are all important—they all indicate null hypotheses and the limited implications scientists are willing to draw from such findings, rather than the sweeping claims headlines may often suggest. To quote one of the researchers in this case, "This discovery takes us *a step closer* to understanding the composition of the core of our sun"—nothing ghostly, and perhaps less sweeping an origin story than an "engine of the universe"; building blocks would be more like it.[4] It is *not* science denial to believe that the headline misrepresents these truths, and I'm passionately convinced that promoting headlines like this (and by promoting, I mean clicking on them and sharing them) dehumanizes scientists and doesn't truly honor their labor-intensive hours (it implies overnight discoveries, for one thing) or the very careful, nuanced nature of the claims they make (by implying these scientists have made bigger or more sweeping claims than they have, for another). *So what?* I hear you saying. I'm just being an annoying literature professor getting on everyone's case about a few word choices. What's the real fallout of any of this? Well,

LESSON 18:
There is no "real" world except what we make.

Okay, I'll admit that I'm being just a little bit purposely annoyingly professorial there. But this concept is something I teach my students nearly every semester, and in nearly every course, whether I'm teaching Medical Humanities or Victorian Literature. Just like Shapin's overly long book title, I constantly teach my students that concepts like "truth" and "fact" are only what we make of them. I learned this distinction the hard way when I dropped out of my psychology pro-

---

4 Ibid.

gram after learning that statistics can only help us interpret chaotic human dynamics—they don't, in fact, quantify them. They take non-numerical data and turn it into numbers that we must then interpret back to non-numerical meaning. There's no shortcut around that part, and humans differ greatly on how they interpret things. The examples of this are endless. Recall from chapter 5 that we could have technically visually seen germs as early as 1670, but for whatever reason, humans weren't ready to interpret that concept as such yet. Or better yet, here's one of my favorite examples to use in teaching this concept of the fluidity of facts. You were probably taught in high school biology the fact that maternal age correlated with chances of conceiving a pregnancy with Down syndrome. The wisdom here was that a woman's eggs are preformed from the moment she herself is conceived, and so it's only logical that their integrity degrades over time. Only in 2002 did someone think to study whether paternal age also correlated with this—and it turns out that it does.[5] Not only eggs degrade when they sit around but sperm, which are produced daily throughout a man's life, are also subject to more frequent mutations and less meticulous checks and balances on such mutations as a man ages. What we see depends on what we look for (my favorite quote for years now, from John Lubbock, a nineteenth-century public figure), and for decades, humanity had been too prone to consider women's ova as "overstocked inventory" subject to deterioration because of age. The result? We missed a whole set of other factors at play in the equation![6]

What is "true" is only defined by how we interpret the world around us, and when we lose sight of that through a problematic faith

5   Method R. Kazaura and Rolv T. Lie, "Down's Syndrome and Paternal Age in Norway," *Pediatric and Perinatal Epidemiology* 16, no. 4 (October 2002): 314–19. This is one of the earliest, but there are others confirming such findings since then.

6   Emily Martin, *Woman in the Body: A Cultural Analysis of Reproduction* (Boston: Beacon, 1987), 49.

in science as a monolithic entity—that is, when we treat science as some sort of Objective Truth Machine spitting facts at us—the repercussions are widespread. For instance, as Molly Fischer notes in her long-form journalism piece "Maybe It's Lyme," it very well may be that chronic pain diagnoses like chronic Lyme disease are the symptom of a society so sickened by overreliance on scientific evidence that we cannot allow for inexplicable pain. What if conditions like this were the result of a very human need for affirmation and validation in a society that simply isn't going to validate experiences that cannot be medically explained or seen under a microscope? As Fischer explains, "Doctors who suggested a psychiatric basis for symptoms . . . [are] understood to translate directly as *All in your head, so get over it.*"[7]

But why do we have a society that refuses to value and affirm things, even if they are in our heads? Our brains, our minds, our hearts, and our feelings are an integral part of us. Fischer continues, "There seemed to exist no acknowledgment that a patient in the grip of a major depressive episode might be unable to think straight, unable to move, unable to get out of bed—nor that telling such a patient to just snap out of it would be as useless as telling a flu patient to try having less of a fever."[8]

The important point to make here is that while doctors are certainly at times responsible for ignoring the claims of the mind, we laypeople are also responsible for buying into this attitude. Instead of resisting such emphasis on the purely biological, we rush—as Fischer has shown, and as I have long suspected as well—to validate our experiences via the commonly accepted biological explanations. Depression won't be affirmed or cared for? Okay, then I'll seek a physical

---

7   Molly Fischer, "Maybe It's Lyme: What Happens When Illness Becomes an Identity," *Cut: New York*, July 24, 2019, www.thecut.com/2019/07/what-happens -when-lyme-disease-becomes-an-identity.html.

8   Ibid.

explanation for my pain and suffering. Of course, these dynamics aren't consciously *chosen*—it's not that people are faking or lying about what they believe is happening to them. Instead, it's that we can't even begin to see through the cultural zeitgeist that we live in. (Sit tight! More on this in just a sec!) We have to be able to slowly remove the problematic biases we hold about science as "Truth" and bodies as "Only Biological" if we are ever to slowly, slowly inch toward a society that can hold depression and anxiety as much in its heart as it does physical ailments. Such a view would recognize, for instance, both Lyme disease and depression as affecting the intertwined dynamics of the *connected, holistic* body-mind, which are never, in fact, separate. It would accept that death and life are part of a continuum, as are sickness and health—never discrete states existing in binary opposition to one another. Letting go of this seeming safety net of Science as Truth would not harm us. Far from it, in fact. It would *help* people get the answers they seek, and it would help doctors better target treatments for patients, while relieving physicians of the pressure to prescribe and treat in particular ways.

If we simply rush to champion what "Science the Great" proclaims as fact instead of carefully considering how those facts are made, we end up putting science to problematic ends, like ceaseless games of whack-a-mole with germs, games that are in fact harmful, not to mention futile. And such games have real-world consequences on people's lives, not just in the microscopic sense of sanitation theater but also in regard to how we handle those who are sick, as we will see in the next chapters.

7

AN ETHICS DEBATE
FOR THE AGES

American Individualism and the
Dilemma of the Healthy Carrier

1906[1]

Imagine this: You are a lecturer of English at a midsize university. In this day of precarity and fading job markets, you feel fortunate to have a renewable contract and health insurance. Perhaps it's this gratitude-guilt that keeps you, more often than not, uncomplaining about your rather overwhelming teaching load and the paltry pay. You're better off than some, in other words, but you work hard. One day, you're typing at your computer in your (shared) office, enjoying the spring sunshine that has just begun to usher out the winter gloom. In spite of the fact that you're technically working through lunch,

---

1 A version of this chapter was previously published in *American Literature* 92 (2020): 737–43. We appreciate their permission to use it here.

you're trying, as best you can, to take a breather between courses when a man storms into your office. He seems . . . official-looking, but a bit harried. Before you can ask what he's doing there, he announces that you, while seemingly healthy, are in fact killing people around you in great numbers with a disease you don't know you have (you vaguely recall hearing about some outbreaks around the country). He claims that he's verified this information with a newfangled form of viral-genotyping software you've never heard of. He tells you it is crucial that you quit your job—*today*—or risk killing more people. He threatens you with forced quarantine if you don't oblige.

What is the ethical choice for you to make as an employee who needs income, and what's more, as a human being who might feel violated by these very suggestions? What's the ethical choice for the official who has discovered this information? Can he, ethically, turn a blind eye to what he's discovered? There's no easy answer here.

This dilemma of conflicting rights that pit an individual's right to informed consent against broader public needs is at least three centuries old. In the 1720s, vaccination debates were often cast as the rights of the individual to deny treatment and/or the necessity of consent for any medical interventions versus the rights of the public to avoid encountering preventable diseases in their community. Like so many public health ethics debates, the question is generally framed as being less about who is "correct" and more about whose civil liberties take precedence when two sets of stakeholders' rights are mutually exclusive and in direct conflict. This is indeed the case. However, as I will show, it's difficult to persuade people about rights when they fundamentally disagree about the lived realities defining these rights. The healthy carrier narrative makes this abundantly clear, and additionally offers a potential means of bridging gaps between ethical obligations on one hand and effective public health communication on the other. The key to bridging these gaps effectively is understanding that

Lesson 19: Public health ethics are a question of personal liberties versus shared rights, but they are first a question of personal versus shared realities.

Lesson 20: You need to know about the socio-scientific discursive cycle.

Lesson 21: In which I discuss German ghosts.

Although the novel coronavirus is more frequently framed as having a long incubation period, this period is in fact *so* long, and the majority of the infected *so mildly* ill, that conceptually, if not scientifically, COVID-19 at least acts like other diseases with healthy carriers. In fact, diseases like this become pandemics much more readily than others. Highly virulent diseases such as the seasonal flu and Ebola tend to be quite visible and therefore more easily avoidable. Conversely, by mid-March 2020, it became apparent that COVID-19 was primarily spread by people who were not yet manifesting symptoms or who might never know they had been ill with the novel coronavirus at all. One by one, countries around the world began issuing stay-at-home orders, the only way to feasibly wait out the virus in a world where anyone could be invisibly carrying a disease. However, people across the planet have struggled with the concept that they must limit their personal activities because of something that isn't, apparently, currently affecting them.

This tension has been thrown into even sharper relief in the United States, a nation with a highly individualistic culture. Crisis-care ethics hold that in times of public health emergencies, health work shifts from a focus on individual needs to a focus on the public's needs.[2]

---

2   Nancy Berlinger et al., "Ethical Framework for Health Care Institutions Responding to Novel Coronavirus SARS-CoV-2 (COVID-19)," Hastings Center, March 16, 2020.

In response to the 2020 COVID-19 pandemic, the Hastings Center explains: "Clinical care is patient-centered, with the ethical course of action aligned, as far as possible, with the preferences and values of the individual patient. Public health practice aims to promote the health of the population by minimizing morbidity and mortality through the prudent use of resources and strategies. Ensuring the health of the population, especially in an emergency, can require limitations on individual rights and preferences."[3]

But America was built on a stubborn skepticism when it comes to submitting to external authorities, especially where it concerns limitations on individual liberties. Thus, the conflict over whose rights matter most has been hard-fought in America, a country where a large number of people still espouse states' rights.

The case study of Mary Mallon, or Typhoid Mary as she is more well known, elucidates the dilemma of the healthy carrier situation quite well.[4] In 1907, Mallon, an Irish immigrant living in New York City, was working as a cook for a local family when a public health official, Dr. George Soper, swooped into her place of employment, pronounced that she was killing those around her with typhoid fever, and demanded a sample of her fecal matter. Mallon shooed him away with a carving fork. Relentless, Soper soon returned. This time Mallon hid. She later absconded from the area completely, finding work under an assumed name. To this day, aside from some revisionist histories that are generally scholarly texts, Mallon is often invoked in popular public

---

3 Ibid., 2.

4 In this recounting of Mary Mallon's experiences, I draw upon both Priscilla Wald, *Contagious: Cultures, Carriers, and the Outbreak Narrative* (Durham, NC: Duke University Press, 2008); and Judith Leavitt, *Typhoid Mary: Captive to the Public Health* (New York: Beacon, 1996). Indeed, Wald notes that the competition between social needs and individual rights in a time of "growing individualism" was always at the heart of the healthy carrier narrative (70).

memory as a selfish and irresponsible woman who didn't care that she was killing others. I, however, tend to see her more in line with recent historical revisions as someone who, in just a decade or so after germ theory became widely accepted as scientific fact, may or may not have been able to *believe* what Soper was telling her. (For lengthier studies of Mallon's history, see Priscilla Wald's *Contagious: Cultures, Carriers, and the Outbreak Narrative* and Judith Leavitt's *Typhoid Mary: Captive to the Public Health*.) To Mary's knowledge, she had never had typhoid, so the new theory of a so-called healthy carrier, justified by the fairly new science of germ theory, may have understandably seemed preposterous to her. I imagine she might have been justly horrified that a man had stormed into her place of employment demanding to look at the contents of her chamber pot. Victorian decorum would have only heightened what even today would be seen as a rather gross violation of one's privacy and workspace.

Yet, from what we can tell, it's likely that Soper was right. Mallon does seem to have been—for all the historical documents can attest (and there are, of course, some limitations to such records)—a healthy carrier of typhoid fever, and her job as a cook was the most dangerous form of employment she could have had with her condition, for touching food with potentially contaminated hands spread the disease readily. Soper ordered Mallon to stop working as a cook, but this sort of job was quite well paying (relatively speaking) for a first-generation Irish immigrant. Racial prejudices at the time were high against the Irish American population, leaving few options for them. Mallon kept working as a cook under an assumed name, where Soper eventually found her and consigned her to quarantine for most of the rest of her life. However, while this last fact might seem to stack the deck in favor of Soper's righteousness, the historical record indicates that Mallon's quarantine-imprisonment was virtually unprecedented either before or after. Many other healthy carriers were identified who then disappeared from the public registers. These were rarely tracked down, and when they were, they were usually let off lightly. As Wald and Leavitt point out, it's difficult to discern exactly why Mallon was confined because of her healthy carrier status when others were not.

To some extent, of course, her nationality and sex may explain these facts. Beyond this, it is cheaper and simpler to pinpoint one "villain" to neutralize than to invest in preventive public health infrastructures. It is cheaper and simpler still (for the state, at least) to promote a national ideology that upholds individual responsibility (rather than government-funded social systems) for cleanliness and hygiene. Indeed, in this period, "social welfare was the responsibility of individuals."[5] Making an example of Mallon promoted the idea of public health progress while avoiding the necessity for larger state investments, as well as side-stepping more nuanced ethical issues inherent to the case.

These ethical considerations are thorny indeed: if Mallon truly refused to stop working as a cook, the rights of the public to be protected from her might have taken preeminence. Typhoid was indeed sporadically epidemic at the time, and so crisis-care ethics would suggest protection of the public over her individual rights. However, in an existential sense, if Mallon truly didn't believe Soper's claims (which used cutting-edge, and possibly confusing, evidence), was she therefore morally obligated to obey his demands? Such a question perhaps exceeds the realm of public health crisis ethics. Yet it is worth considering in order to develop a more effective means of promoting compliance with public health recommendations in the future. Outside of academic texts, Mallon has mostly been portrayed as someone who did not *care* that she was infecting others. How does the ethical scale shift if we suppose that she *cared* but did not *believe*? This leads us to the lesson that

---

5 Wald, *Contagious*, 72.

LESSON 19:

Public health ethics are a question of personal liberties versus shared rights, but they are first a question of personal versus shared realities.

This last question yields particular insight into the issue plaguing America today: we might portray those who oppose social distancing as MAGA-hat-wearing, gun-toting individualists who are unconcerned with the public good, but what if the healthy carrier narrative is one that fundamentally pits not only two sets of rights but also two sets of *lived realities*—embodied realities, at that—against one another? For the moment, let's set aside the important issue of economic realities discussed in earlier chapters, issues affecting those who cannot live without the income that leaving their house provides. What of those who simply cannot believe that the evidence of their own individual senses—their own perception of their own bodies—should take a back seat to scientific data? Aside from being an ethical dilemma, this is also a public health and scientific communication dilemma of great import to future generations, foreshadowed by the healthy carrier experience of Mary Mallon. Indeed, beginning with Mallon's case, public health expectations began to "introduce . . . experts, such as the epidemiologist, who would serve as a mediating role between citizens and the state," and whose authority individual(istic) Americans were asked to substitute for their own perceptions of their bodies and the environment.[6]

America is the land of boot-strapping individualism, and that mindset has long extended to expectations that good American citizens look out for their own health (think about the media campaigns you see to go get mammograms or to know the signs of a stroke).

---

6   Ibid., 70.

Ironically, this grassroots method of trying to keep a large population healthy through self-management and self-monitoring leads us to a predicament in which we suddenly need everyone to do the *same thing* for public health reasons. First, we're asking a population steeped in individualistic culture to concern itself with the public good—for public rights to supersede individual rights, that is. But second and just as important, we're asking individuals to believe in a publicly defined reality and not in a personally informed one. In short, we're asking Americans to suddenly stop doing everything that we generally ask them to do in regard to public health (look after your own body, monitor your own symptoms) and instead urging an about-face (do things to protect other people's bodies, and stop assuming you know what your own body is "telling you").[7]

In fact, we're doing more than this: we're asking individuals to *deny* a personally informed reality of a self, substituting in its place aggregated data about the global public. This is a tall order, to say the least. It's a tension that is more than simply assuming that America, as a whole, cares too little for the public good (as I admittedly often do—I make no exceptions for myself). Science communication and public health ethics can be helpfully informed through the evolving legacy of the healthy carrier narrative, which demonstrates that we must think *like* those we wish to influence (**Lessons 10 and 11**), however much we may want to lament their perceived lack of ethical concern for the common good.

I began this chapter with a thought experiment, which I hope serves this purpose. However, any number of scenarios could be substituted, as long as they involve being confronted with an urgent request to deeply believe anything that seems fundamentally untrue to you. For me, being asked to believe—at peril of the end of the world—

---

7 In general, I'm happy to lump the Western first world together, but as far as individualistic gumption goes, I think America stands a bit apart here.

that global warming is *not* happening serves the purpose. Even nearer to the mark would be examples that pit (as the novel coronavirus and shelter-in-place orders have) individual bodily sensations against some broader, ambiguous set of data and for a broader cause. What if you were told that your chronic headaches were imaginary? This might be the sort of analogous example that de-escalates the intensity of the debates over lockdowns for possibly healthy carriers brought up in 2020, but it lacks urgency. What if you were told not only that your headaches were imaginary but also that you *must* believe they don't exist for the benefit of your neighbor, who needs your medication (as there's a shortage in this imagined scenario)? The neighbor, you're told, won't accept the medicine from you if you're actually ill, so it's imperative that you disbelieve your own pain to save your neighbor's life (for the sake of argument, let's say that this medicine treats multiple things, since the stakes are different for asymptomatic COVID-19 carriers than for those who become dangerously ill). That would be a hard pill to swallow (or to let your neighbor swallow while you sat in pain).

And remember, reality is only what we make it (**Lesson 18**), which brings me to what my students, at least, always tell me is the most useful thing I ever teach them. Enter

LESSON 20:
You need to know about the socio-scientific discursive cycle.
(DON'T LET THE FANCY LANGUAGE FOOL YOU.
YOU NEED TO READ THIS.)

Without naming it directly, I've been referring to the socio-scientific discursive cycle (let's nickname her the SSDC) in many parts of this book—when talking about death culture, when explaining how germ theory made us want to clean far too much, and when discussing why we humans are far too willing to believe in cure-alls. The SSDC shapes how we view our world, what becomes "real" to us, and how the values we have transform into tangible practices.

Simply put, the SSDC is how science and society are constantly influencing each other. It's my term for the process by which scientific language influences the way we see the world and how this worldview cycles back to inform the creation of science (this includes the questions scientists think to ask, the funding different topics are allocated, and how research methodology is structured). It's a cousin concept to **Lesson 18**, where I discussed our tendency to value physical over mental pain, and the way we have constructed research of certain health conditions.

A quick example will help here. Long before germ theory existed to prove that contagious disease germs were spread by human vectors, people very readily acknowledged that humans can "contaminate" one another's thinking, morals, and behavior. The idea of the contagious influence of knowledge (though they didn't always use that word) vastly predates any scientific framework of contagion. As I mentioned in chapter 5, Laura Otis has demonstrated that the microscopes capable of seeing disease germs existed at least a century before germ cells were explained by scientists as such. Eventually, for whatever reason (and there are many explanations for this that I won't get into here; I suggest Otis, as summarized in chapter 5, if you're curious), scientists *were* able to conceive of the contaminating nature of the particles they had always seen under the microscopes, influenced by the world they could see macroscopically around them. If humans can "infect" one another's thinking, might not these microscopic particles spread through their own networks and infect us with disease?

Enter the next social/conceptual step of the cycle, in which humans start to see more and more structures in the world as defined by webs of connectivity. It's a small wonder, then, that by the 1990s, the World Wide Web was described *and*—this is important—*designed* to be a connective network tying people to one another. This technological discourse was germinated through centuries of seeing the world through frameworks of connection, networks, and contagion. It's no coincidence, in other words, that we call computer viruses *viruses*. But my point is that it doesn't stop at language—the very concept of a computer virus, something that invades and then infects the host by forcing it to replicate its own body, could not have existed in a computer coder's mind if the concept of viruses as biological organisms did not already exist. And to take it further, it's highly likely that our concept of viruses as invading organisms that take over and force replication of themselves is a way of explaining infection that was only possible to us based on already existing ways of thinking about the world in terms of power, colonization, and invasion (I direct the reader to Otis, Servitje, and Sudan for more about these concepts).

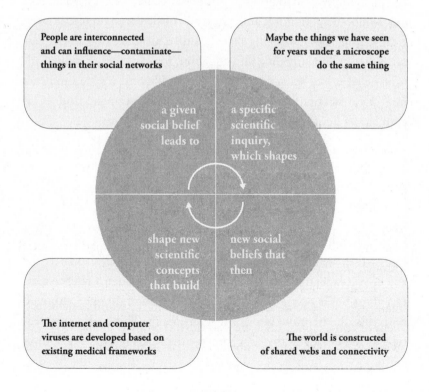

People are interconnected and can influence—contaminate—things in their social networks

Maybe the things we have seen for years under a microscope do the same thing

a given social belief leads to

a specific scientific inquiry, which shapes

shape new scientific concepts that build

new social beliefs that then

The internet and computer viruses are developed based on existing medical frameworks

The world is constructed of shared webs and connectivity

A great deal of my public and academic work has lamented a lack of community-minded goals in modern Western society, but the SSDC is a self-perpetuating machine, so I'll be the first to admit that I'm less certain how to solve the problem of differing realities (as opposed to differing values). In general, the era of "fake news" as a concept has sowed a tendency to doubt not just expertise but also claims to reality on the whole. It seems difficult, despairingly impossible even, to ever find common ground when no one can agree on what the "ground" is to begin with. This may be one of the most important revelations COVID-19 has given us: we have come to a point of such hyperpolarization in the Western world that we deny that we have *any* shared realities. There is no news or fact we can agree on, period.

Not this disease. Not here. Not in my body. I feel fine.

It is simply hard to break free from our belief in the experiences of our own bodies, but this is an even greater difficulty to overcome when we're talking about changing shared cultural attitudes (like the American belief in bootstrapping individualism, for instance). A shared cultural belief is like being trapped in an invisible box. It's hard to break free, of course, but first you have to realize you're trapped, and this is even harder because you can't see the box to begin with.

LESSON 21:
In which I discuss German ghosts.

In my discipline, we affectionately refer to this sort of box as a *zeitgeist*, which literally translates into "time ghost." Unfortunately for any of you expecting spooky surprises, a zeitgeist doesn't refer to a literal ghost but is better understood as "the spirit of the age," although even this doesn't quite pin down its meaning. Think of any stereotype of any decade in the last century—the Roaring Twenties, Flower

Power of the sixties—any of these could certainly be said to illustrate the zeitgeist of that era. But zeitgeists can also be more specific than this, and it's the SSDC that ends up developing a decent portion of our zeitgeists, the sorts of zeitgeist that can be doubly hard to see outside of because they define more than just lifestyle practices. They define everything we think we know about our collective identities and our collective realities.

Of relevance here is the zeitgeist of "I know best about my body." It's a lesson we teach people from almost before they can talk: "You know your body," "Listen to your body," and so forth. And while these are great truisms to teach our children about consent and empowerment as they grow older, they do come with blinders as they become our entire culture's zeitgeist. How can we really expect people to do a 180 on this logic all of a sudden in 2021? Is it really reasonable to expect people to suddenly ignore the evidence of their bodily sensations because we say they should now, after years of a different zeitgeist reigning supreme? Again—and #sorrynotsorry if I sound like a broken record here—it would be more productive of us to ask for the broad cultural reasons that people resist such mandates, rather than scolding individuals for not conforming. Only then, I think, can we slowly begin to change our collective zeitgeists to those that encourage ownership and empowerment of our own bodies and *also* add in a healthy dose of "Sometimes the body is silent" or "Trust one's own body in collaboration with trusted experts" or something of the like. Ironically enough, the very denial of any shared realities that I mentioned in **Lesson 20** is its own zeitgeist that has been gaining momentum for the last five years or so. I worry that this only allows the virus—or any other pathogen in our future—a foothold. Our divisions are their smorgasbord. How can we plan or strategize if we can't agree that we need to plan or strategize to begin with? This is one of the biggest hurdles we'll need to overcome to ensure humanity's long-term survival. It's possibly one of the most terrifying threats to humanity that I've seen in my lifetime—for if our only shared belief is that there are no shared beliefs, where do we go from there?

Zeitgeists can and do change over time, but only with the small actions of many people working to change them. Think about movements like #MeToo and MAGA. The collective actions of many individual people created those changes to the way we think about our world. Maybe more women than we think really are assaulted. Was America great before? Now you've got someone wondering. In a way, you could say that zeitgeists themselves are contagious, but they must be conscientiously cultivated and nurtured to grow in the direction we want or need them to, like so many bacteria in a petri dish. Ghostbusters can't help us here, and criticizing one person is going to do no good against a whole era full of time-ghosts.

———

As we can see from Mary Mallon, and from the earlier vaccination debates, issues of conflicting rights can get heated, indeed. But even Mallon eventually seemed to accept that her confinement was in the public's best interest, capitulating to public *rights* because she had eventually accepted some part of the public *reality* presented to her by germ-theory science. Indeed, the archival evidence indicates that she sent her fecal samples out for independent lab investigation, suggesting that she ultimately recognized the validity of Soper's science- and germ theory–based reasoning, even if she was skeptical about its claims about specific germs in her specific body. How much faster might this have occurred if they could have communicated better, learned alongside each other, and brainstormed solutions together?

Perhaps it does come back to valuing community, after all. Recent studies in science communication have suggested what I've sketched out in this chapter: that scientific literacy is not the variable that determines whether or not a group will accept the reality of a public health issue like vaccination or global warming; social groups are. While those individuals tested demonstrated a surprising ability to factually interpret scientific findings, they tended to eventually revert to in-group thinking about the issue, siding with whatever their main social group already believed.[8] We humans are social, after all. Our social nature is why solitary confinement is potentially a human rights violation, why just about *all of us* wish we weren't having to stay home during the COVID crisis, why we all cling to Zoom get-togethers—even as we dread another second of Zoom meetings—why children yell at one another across balconies, starved for the sound of another child's voice. We all do the same dance of retreating to our social safety spaces. And if our "safe" social group told us that our experience during the coronavirus pandemic was a lie? Well, it seems we'd be more likely to believe our friends than science, because, as I've argued elsewhere,[9] and as Matthew Arnold famously proclaimed in his lyrical poem "Dover Beach," in times of desperate calamity, all we humans really have is one another. I have no answer to this twisted dilemma that the healthy carrier narrative, via the vehicle of COVID-19, has presented to us in the United States, but understanding the dilemma rightly is surely important. In ethics, we make algorithms. But humans are not algorithms. And perhaps understanding that will be a meaningful first step toward bridging the gaps hyperpolarized politics have rent in our world. Doing so matters, because as I said in the anti-chapter, all we have in the face of

---

8   Dan Kahan, "Fixing the Communications Failure," *Nature* 463 (2010): 296–97.

9   In *Kept from All Contagion*.

calamity is our social support networks. Which is why Arnold cries out in this poem, "let us be true to one another." For

> *The world, which seems*
> *To lie before us like a land of dreams,*
> *So various, so beautiful, so new,*
> *Hath really neither joy, nor love, nor light,*
> *Nor certitude, nor peace, nor help for pain;*
> *And we are here as on a darkling plain*
> *Swept with confused alarms of struggle and flight,*
> *Where ignorant armies clash by night.*[10]

---

10   Matthew Arnold, "Dover Beach," 1867.

8

THE KIDS ARE NOT ALL RIGHT

When Diseases Like the 1918
Influenza Pandemic Take the Young

=====

1918

Try to recall the last time you imagined an orphanage.

Come on, we've all done it. If the Victorians left us nothing else, they left us a series of oddly vivid images of abandoned, family-less children in workhouses and cobblestoned alleyways.

I cannot possibly be the only parent who has taught her toddlers to hold up empty cereal bowls, look plaintively up at the nearest adult, and whimper, "Please, sir, I want some more." Even if you don't know that this famous line comes from Charles Dickens's novel *Oliver Twist*, chances are you're familiar with the quote itself. Orphans and orphanages are an idea so ingrained in our cultural consciousness that the image is still used when we think of things like international adoptions or relief agencies.

So, seriously. Stop for a second and think of an orphanage.

Most of us probably imagine a barren room, serving as little more than a baby warehouse for tragically unwanted living goods. The smells of unchanged diapers, the unending cries of hundreds of needy babies . . .

Except, wait—that's not right. Do you know the creepiest thing about actual orphanages? The babies don't cry. At all.

Anyone who has seen babies in really any setting in which their basic needs are at least minimally met may think that babies never stop crying, but ironically it's babies whose needs *are* met that cry. Like any creature designed to evolve and cling to survival with a vise grip, infants can and do simply give up if their cries go unheard for long enough. Their primal resource management systems are sophisticated enough to know when energy output (crying) is not being compensated with resource input (food), and they simply stop wasting precious calories with their cries.

Which brings me to my point: You've probably been imagining orphanages wrong. And this now makes your reimagining of orphanages somehow creepier, right? That's because we know that babies *should* cry. Their cries are admittedly annoying, but their silence is unnatural. It bespeaks a psychic wound of some kind that—even if you hadn't read all this—you'd instinctively *know* wasn't right. Babies cry. It's what they do. It's annoying, but it's the design of babies.

So, you're probably wondering why I'm beginning a chapter on the 1918 influenza pandemic with a thought experiment on orphanages. It's an effort to demonstrate that we have certain expectations about various phases of life, particularly infancy through young adulthood. By the time we in the West reach thirty or forty, we're generally an undifferentiated mass of "middle-aged [people] who buy hamburger meat and toilet paper on sale," to quote the Norwegian minister of health, Bent Høie.[1] The Youth, as I sometimes jokingly call them, have much more character in each of their various life phases

---

1   Translated by Rachel Petersen.

and are much more readily distinguishable by these defining characteristics. And as much as those of us in our thirties and forties like to
shake our fists at the world around us, my aim in this chapter is to
convince you, dear reader, that you'd find it much weirder without
the occasional beer pong party that you notice on a drive through
your local college district (yes, this is absolutely a nod to the house
near mine). Babies cry. Little kids play with each other. Teenagers are
emotional and angsty. College-aged kids have wild parties. Yes, it can
be frustrating and annoying to us boring, ground-beef-sale Old Tim-
ers, but these things define the cycles of life that make our world seem
normal. These phase-of-life signals help us *feel* the machinations of the
world spinning onward. They make us *sense palpably* that we are surrounded by a population properly going through their growth cycles,
completing the proverbial Circle of Life.

Perhaps none of anything I've written here needs to be stated anymore, because if nothing else, the COVID-19 pandemic has left all of
us starkly aware of the things we should have been appreciating but
had begun to take for granted: live theater and music, the drudgery of
school drop-off and pickup, and, yes, even the loud college parties we
roll our eyes at.

And yet, I think it matters precisely *how* we interpret this eerie
emptiness. It doesn't just point to the COVID-19 pandemic generally.
It points to very specific losses suffered by very specific people in very
specific ways, ways that will ultimately impact all of us. It points to a
New Lost Generation. If we want to save a generation on the brink, we
need to learn from our most recently threatened generation, those who
lived through the 1918 influenza pandemic. Their encounters with
pandemic disease—the most modern evidence of such we have—teach
us that

**Lesson 22: We were prepared. We just weren't prepared to
be prepared.**

Lesson 23:   The kids are not all right.

**Lesson 24:   The fallout already existed—it was just more
                convenient to ignore.**

A note to readers before we dive in: like Defoe's literary wisdom, the 1918 influenza pandemic has much to offer us in our modern day. Whereas Defoe provides an important view of how societies reacted to plagues in an era we can access only through archives, some researchers alive today have had the ability to actually interview survivors of the 1918 pandemic and learn from them. These lived experiences are vital and their cultural contexts are very similar to our own, both relatively speaking and when compared against the whole of human history. I believe these lived experiences are so important for us to learn from that in this chapter I've included not only the usual lessons and anecdotes found in other chapters but also specific warnings and takeaways from survivors that I think can help us survive as well.

In general, young men and women alike were victims of that terrible disease, in numbers never seen before. One survivor, James Pharis, would later recount that the "people that die[d] [were] the very stoutest of people." He recalled having conversations with friends who would be dead the next day and added that people would just suddenly drop dead while they were walking.[2] What was perhaps most frightening is that never before had anyone seen a disease wipe out the middle of the life cycle—those in their twenties, thirties, and forties—as aggressively as the 1918 influenza pandemic. And while no one ever liked to see *anyone* die, there was something about seeing young mothers and fathers or college-aged

---

2   Interview with James and Nannie Pharis, oral narrative, *Going Viral: Impact and Implications of the 1918 Flu Pandemic*, Southern Oral History Program, University of North Carolina Libraries, January 8, 1979.

kids die so suddenly and in such rampant numbers that made this pandemic all the more horrifying. It just didn't adhere to the normal cycles of life—or death. In fact, no pandemic in written history has wiped out as many people as the 1918 flu pandemic. Not COVID-19. Not the Black Plague. No disease in recorded history has ever been so deadly in such quick bursts. And its horrors were increased because people saw those who were traditionally seen as the strongest, the most impervious to disease, falling in droves. It was the silent orphanage writ large, and the world grew eerily quiet as more and more young people died.

Sparks Memorial Hospital
Fort Smith, Arkansas
1915[3]

Alice Mikel cocked her head as far as she could to the right and hitched her right shoulder up to her ear. She rotated her head a little back and forth, coming as close as she could to scratching the terrible itch that she had from the pins holding up her outdated Gibson Girl hairdo—part of the dress code. She frowned and then straightened back up, mentally preparing herself to continue her duties. Straightening her crisp, pink uniform, its white-aproned bib crossed jauntily in the back, she proceeded down the hallways of the hospital. In spite of the awful regulation hairstyle, the job was a good one. There were few jobs for women in general, and if you were accepted for nursing training, sup-

---

3 Because the date that Alice joined the nursing school is, as far as I can tell, unrecorded, this may have occurred as late as 1916. However, given that she mentions the outbreak of World War I while she was a nurse, it's more likely to have been an earlier date in 1915.

plies and board were covered. It was a decent way to get on in the world if you didn't want to get married right away, and Alice didn't. "No one was gonna marry me," she'd later say saucily at the age of 105 (although she did eventually get married three times).[4]

"Our boys aren't getting the proper treatment . . ." Alice's ears perked up as she approached a room where a woman was speaking to a group of nursing students. The war was on everyone's minds, of course, and everyone wanted to help however they could. For women in particular, the "how" of that equation was a puzzler. What could a woman do in war?

"Well, I'm recruiting for the Red Cross. When you graduate, I hope . . . that you join the Red Cross and be a Red Cross Nurse."

They all said yes.

Camp Pike
Little Rock, Arkansas
1918

By this time, Alice had exchanged her alluring pink uniform for a plain blue one—still with the jaunty cross-tied back. The differences between Sparks Memorial and Camp Pike were as stark as her uniform change: from the clean white of the hospital to the barracks full of the sick, Alice, who had signed up to be in the thick of World War I, found to her surprise that she had also enlisted to be in the middle of the 1918 influenza pandemic. At 105 years old, she could still vividly recall a night when the morgue was too full of bodies to accept more.

---

4 Alice L. Mikel Duffield, *Veterans History Project*, oral narrative, April 22, 2002, https://memory.loc.gov/diglib/vhp/story/loc.natlib.afc2001001.01747/?loclr=bl ogflt.

As they opened the door to place a new body, the overcrowded morgue belched its contents, and a corpse fell nearly on top of them. One of the orderlies, she said, a grown man, screamed that he couldn't take it anymore.[5]

Alice looked out at the road, trying not to let his screams infect her with panic. People said the outbreak started in the camps, and it was hard to deny the possibility as she watched the trucks full of bodies coasting along the road. Back and forth, back and forth they cruised, between the barracks and the morgue of Camp Pike, as if overwhelming death tolls were the most natural thing in the world. It reminded her of the zoetrope she used to play with as a child, a little carousel that she could spin with her hand. Inside was a strip of pictures, one next to the other. When she spun the device, the pictures blurred together and appeared to be moving, but they could only ever represent a short, looping image, *round and round and round.* Her favorite as a child had been one with a devil playing leapfrog over the back of a man—up and down he'd hop, back and forth, like the corpse trucks on the road, heedless of nothing but the onward spin of their loop . . . *round and round and round.*

Barre, Vermont[6]

Ernest looked out his bedroom window. Another funeral procession was plodding down the street below his home to the cemetery. There was nothing to do while he and his whole family were sick other than stare out the window, but even a young boy could tire of the same

---

5   Ibid.

6   Interview with Ernest V. Reynolds, "The Flu Epidemic, 1918," *Vermont History*, March 24, 1988, https://vermonthistory.org/flu-epidemic-1918.

black horses and the same black carriage passing up and down, up and down, day in and day out. He pressed his nose to the glass and watched anyway, though. Back and forth, back and forth, as if the carriage were designed to do nothing else but pace an endless procession. It reminded him of a tin windup toy, going mindlessly forward with jerky but ceaseless momentum. The silence in the town was crushing if he listened to it too closely—it seemed like *everyone* was sick and dying—and it seemed safer to distract himself with the tin toy procession on the road below.

Madrid
Houston County, Alabama[7]

Almost 1,400 miles away in a smaller town than its name suggested, little Edna marched out her front door dutifully. She was ten now, old enough to help, and Mother reckoned that as their family was the only one that had somehow not contracted the awful influenza, it was their duty to help all the neighbors.

"Wait!"

Edna turned back upon hearing her mother's voice. She squinted as she saw the thin fabric waving in the air. *Oh.* She marched back to the door and waited patiently while her mother tied the gauze bandage around her face, so that she didn't catch the flu when she visited her neighbors. Then she was off. She enjoyed the *clink, clink, clink* of the mason jars filled with soup that she carried. Each day, Mother pack-

---

7 Interview with Edna R. Boone, "Pandemic Influenza," Alabama Public Health, March 2007, http://video1.adph.state.al.us/alphtn/pandemic/EdnaBoone/Local /transcript_ednaboone.pdf.

aged them for Edna to drop off on the neighbors' porches. She relished feeling important as she stayed up late, making sure the hot water reservoir in the stove was replenished as Mother sterilized the jars over and over each night, then filled them with more soup. The next morning, Edna would dutifully carry these labor-intensive meals back and forth to the neighbors on repeat, like a slowly looping zoetrope, or a very tired windup tin soldier, keeping time with the rhythmic grind of her gears.

Conover, North Carolina[8]

Glenn listened to the rhythmic chant by which he'd come to define his days.

"Ya in there?" It was like a repeated refrain of a song, circling round and round his mind. It was a kind way the neighbors had of making sure their friends were still alive, while avoiding the influenza themselves. People would pop by, peer in the windows, and gently call, "Ya in there?" It was certainly a pleasanter turn of phrase than "Did you die last night?" His father went to the window and said, "We're all right in here." Like the call and counter-call of two birds, whistled back and forth on the breeze, notes invisibly looping upward—a resounding medley of a community waiting out death.

---

8 Interview with Gladys and Glenn Hollar, *Going Viral: Impact and Implications of the 1918 Flu Pandemic*, Southern Oral History Program, University of North Carolina Libraries, February 26, 1980, https://exhibits.lib.unc.edu/exhibits/show /going-viral/oral-histories.

Philadelphia, Pennsylvania[9]

There was nowhere to put them, all the dead people. "They died in piles," she'd later say.[10] The grave diggers themselves were dead or dying, and so were the undertakers and the coffin makers. Mama said the woman down the street had begged the wagon to wait while she fetched a macaroni box to put her seven-year-old son's body in (at the time, pasta came in large wooden crates that could hold twenty pounds each).[11] At least he wasn't carted away in just a sheet. People offered boards from their very houses to help make coffins for their neighbors.[12] And so little Louise just clipped away. There was nothing for it but for families to help themselves, or neighbors to help where they could, and Mother thought it was just awful for a person to lie in an undressed casket—especially the babies. The gentle *snip, snip* of the scissors as she scalloped the edges of lace to put over their coffin was all they could offer to mark the tiny lives, and so the *snip, snip, snip*

---

9   This particular anecdote is a combination of two women's stories: Louise Apuchase of Philadelphia recounted the macaroni box story, and Ninnie Shepherd of Poll's Creek, Kentucky, recalled cutting coffin dressings. To avoid the possible confusion of using Ninnie's name here and Nannie's in the next story, I've opted to use Louise's name but want to credit the oral histories of both women.

10 James and Nannie Pharis interview.

11 Louise Apuchase, George Mason University's Roy Rosenzweig Center for History and New Media, *History Matters* oral history archives, http://historymatters .gmu.edu/d/13/.

12 Credit for this detail goes to an unnamed man from Pettigrew, Arkansas. Quoted by Stephanie Hall in the Library of Congress's *Folklife Today: American Folklife Center and Veteran's History Project*, "Stories from the 1918–1919 Influenza Pandemic from Ethnographic Collections," https://blogs.loc.gov/folklife/2020/04 /stories-influenza-pandemic/.

carried on, pulsating, metallic notes of mourning against the silence.[13] Like the fates clipping off the threads of life, Louise clipped lace to honor death. *Snip, snip, snip.*

Spray, North Carolina[14]

Nannie had never seen so many dead pregnant women, and what she couldn't stop thinking about was how the babies would get out if their mamas were dead. She supposed they just shriveled up together. A young married woman herself, she knew the answer, but she couldn't shake the horror of the image. Entire families were dead. And while the neighbors—if there were any neighbors not sick—would leave groceries, people knew better than to come inside to help nurse patients. The silence was suffocating in the houses of the dying. There were none of the comforting sounds of a friend or family member helping out in another room, the sounds of their movements reassuring you that the world was running along smoothly, and that you'd be running smoothly, too, in no time. There was only the silence of an entire generation of dead young people, and the nightmarish zoetrope of corpse transportation revolving fiendishly outside your window whenever you looked.

———

Some days I worry that our present-day zoetrope is gaining momentum. In just the two months between drafting and revising this manu-

---

13 Interview with Ninnie Shepherd, April 5, 1979, *Frontier Nursing Service Oral History Project*, Louie B. Nunn Center for Oral History, University of Kentucky, https://kentuckyoralhistory.org/ark:/16417/xt7rr49g7c3b.

14 James and Nannie Pharis interview.

script, the death toll in America has skyrocketed—it's worse than it was when we all panicked in March. And yet, we're all so tired. So, this is going to be the second of two times I get avowedly, unashamedly political in this book (the first was in chapter 4 about the Black Lives Matter movement): the presidential administration facing the novel coronavirus in 2020 was prepared, but they weren't prepared to be prepared.

LESSON 22:
We were prepared. We just weren't prepared to be prepared.

In 2007, the CDC collaborated with a group of historians to compile as much data as they could about the 1918 influenza outbreak (sometimes called the Spanish flu, but to avoid xenophobic language, I will refer to it as the former). The CDC's logic was similar to that of this book: in the 1920s and previously, there were no reasonably effective pharmaceutical interventions to help with the flu. There were only behavioral ones, and we needed to understand the effectiveness of those behavioral interventions so that we could be prepared in advance for any future pandemics. The formal analysis of this data was published in the 2007 issue of the *Journal for the American Medical Association*, and in this study the authors call such behavioral methodologies "nonpharmaceutical interventions."[15] Even today, as we saw in 2020, vaccine development takes quite some time. By studying nonpharmaceutical interventions implemented by different cities across America and then statistically analyzing flu trends from those various cities, researchers hoped they could learn how to handle a pandemic

---

15 Howard Markel et al., "Nonpharmaceutical Interventions Implemented by US Cities During the 1918–1919 Influenza Pandemic," *Journal of the American Medical Association* 298 (2007): 644–54.

disease outbreak if and when it next occurred, while we waited for pharmaceutical interventions to be developed. What the study showed is fairly cut-and-dried: enforcing social distancing, wearing masks, and closing schools, implemented as early as possible, were the best means of controlling the disease and preventing "excess death rates." So, there was a plan—a plan that had been specifically developed to help us cope with a pandemic disease outbreak.

But we in the United States didn't use it, or at least we didn't use it early enough. I will admit that the public adoption of mask-wearing was slowed in part by the CDC's changing recommendations. Although I think there are several good reasons why the CDC might have initially said not to wear masks (such as fears that people would hoard them and deprive frontline health workers), they took a real gamble in terms of public confidence when the infection rates trended upward and they shifted their recommendations to support mask-wearing.[16] That being said, in addition to the public reluctance to adopt safety protocols (I outlined some cultural reasons for this reluctance in chapter 7), I do also believe that there was significant responsibility on the part of the executive branch of the federal government that contributed to the slow pandemic response. The 2020 presidential administration was unwilling to actually implement the findings of the 2007 *JAMA* article, findings that had been commissioned for exactly this very time and purpose.

So, we had pragmatically prepared (back in 2007), but we weren't psychologically prepared to execute our practical knowledge. Why? For virtually all of the reasons I've covered in this book so far: fear, denial, and a belief that we're somehow beyond the true reach of infectious disease. These all lead to a misguided belief—a zeitgeist, if you will (**Lesson 21**)—that it can't happen here, to us, right now. All the pragmatic preparation, all the intellectual understanding, all the re-

---

16   This is, of course, simply my opinion. I'm not actually privy to what went into their decision-making about recommendations regarding masks over time.

fined knowledge in the world can't necessarily equip us for psychically handling the fact that we, too, are mortal. That is a deeper psychological preparation, and only careful self-reflection can begin to unstick these problematic beliefs. By doing things such as deeply accepting the truth of our own individual mortality (hey-o, anti-chapter!) and disillusioning ourselves about the possibility of complete risk aversion (**Lessons 6 and 13**), we can begin to contribute our voices to the collective changes we need, like altering our communal zeitgeists (**Lesson 21**).

The wise words of these survivors beg us to remember, to prepare.

Instead, in 2020, having not been prepared to be prepared, we side-stepped one form of a Lost Generation only to find that we created another. Because

LESSON 23:
The kids are not all right.

Yeah, yeah, it's the chapter title, too, but I can't help it. It's the phrase that keeps ringing in my head everywhere I look. Don't get me wrong, the COVID-19 pandemic meant we *had* to shut down schools early in 2020 while we regrouped. But I wonder what our benchmark will be for opening things up again. And I mean an evidence-based benchmark, not simply a choice made because we're tired of being careful. As much as I wish we'd masked up and shut down earlier in America, I have also been increasingly concerned as I watch the goalposts change while reopening. All of a sudden, by April 2020, every like-minded liberal around me seemed to have suddenly awoken to the always-true reality that infectious disease can, does, did, and has always killed us in the "Developed World," too. And just like that, the fears were insurmountable (recall the denial/panic pendulum in **Lesson 6**). What I witnessed both at home

IF YOU COULD HAVE A DO-OVER . . .

What several survivors wished they could tell future generations:[1]

I think the only thing I could suggest . . . is to be aware that it could happen again. Children need to learn about what could happen. . . . The shock wave that sets in when something like this happens kind of stuns people, you know. They go beyond thinking correctly.

—Edna Register Boone, age 100

Everybody would just go to Walmart or all these other places [if a pandemic ever occurred again]. . . . Now people don't stay at home when they're sick. . . . They go spread whatever they got.

—Gurtys Robinson, 97

Go to your doctor, get your medicine, go home, be sure you've got plenty of food, and stay there.

—Annie Laurie Williams, 91

I think people in this day and time need to take more in consideration of [how] diseases are transferred . . . and be informed about them.

—Agnes Gatlin, 100

---

1 Thanks to the Alabama Public Health 1918 Oral History Collection for this set of narratives, and for asking a vital question. Alabama Public Health, *1918 Pandemic Influenza Survivors Share Their Stories*, https://www.alabamapublichealth.gov/pandemicflu/1918-influenza-survivor-stories.html.

and in the nation at large was the initial need to "flatten the curve" (that is, prevent hospitals from being overwhelmed and pushed past their capacity) slide slowly into "no risk is acceptable," and suddenly, things we'd been doing all along—school, for instance—became too risky to us. As you'll remember from **Lessons 7 and 8**, all human connection is contagious, and it always has been, but we were simply willing to take the risk before 2020. I'm not going to debate whether or not COVID-19 is worse than the seasonal flu, mostly because this argument has become too politicized to be useful, but also because I don't think comparative analyses of risk should be the point.

Increasingly, I don't see society focusing on an endpoint but rather leaning into the forever-limbo of whack-a-mole (**Lesson 13**) and total risk elimination (**Lesson 6**). And while we might have avoided a Lost Generation by doing this (although COVID-19 does not attack the young with the verve that the 1918 flu did), I wonder about a Lost Generation of children who have missed out on nearly a year of socialization and learning. My daughter's kindergarten was open in fall 2020, and I elected to send her back, because for me, the risk of her not seeing other children was larger than the risk of COVID-19. That's my personal choice, and I don't ask you to agree with it, but hear me out. Her teacher, Rachel Taasaas, had initially noted some pretty troubling differences in these newly minted kindergarteners after five months of quarantine, compared to what she normally expects to see in a new group of kiddos. Perhaps the most concerning thing that she told me is the children's inability to focus on real human faces, in person, if they aren't projected on a screen. She also noted the children having difficulties with following simple two-step directions, which doesn't sound so bad, until she described what she's seeing further. When asked to do something such as "Put this in the sink, and then go to the book area," the students simply say, "What did you say?"[2] But she has noticed

---

2   Rachel Taasaas, personal communication.

that, if given a pause during which to process, the children realize they have in fact heard and understood the command. This seems to me an awful lot like a computer processing lag, which I'm not entirely sure what to make of.[3] The teacher's theory is pretty simple: a game or an app will repeat things forever if you keep hammering buttons, and so listening to interpersonal communication the first time simply isn't a learned skill for children the way it may have been before COVID-19. Just a little less than a year of remote learning has already deactivated a skill that we have always taken for granted.

Another dire consequence is that doctors everywhere have noted increases in domestic violence, and it's hard to deny that that's a real cost to children who are trapped with their abusers—this phenomenon was even featured in an article by the Health Resources and Services Administration of the US Department of Health and Human Services. *Radiology*, a professional physician's journal, published X-ray evidence of this increase in its August 13, 2020, issue, and the *New York Times* notes the global rise of domestic violence since the lockdowns began. I find it equally troubling that this data has been used by those resisting COVID-19 precautions as much as it has been ignored by those who *support* quarantine. As I've said numerous times in countless ways, it doesn't have to be an either/or solution. If we could, on both sides of these debates, stop digging in our heels and resisting each other's claims for the sake of toeing our party line (that is, retreating to the safety of our social circles, per **Lesson 12**, and only using scientific evidence as it suits us to strengthen our already existing beliefs). Only then might we be able to develop more nuanced solu-

---

3 While at the time of this writing there are very few educational studies that have explored this specific interaction (although many are in the works), UNICEF has documented a concern over early childhood development because of the COVID-19 pandemic. Their assessment can be found at https://data.unicef.org/topic/early-childhood-development/covid-19/.

tions that take precautions for the virus *and* buffer the vulnerable from domestic violence situations.

Regardless, it's likely that none of this is news to you, and you may even feel that I'm rubbing salt in wounds you're all too aware of but don't know how to heal. What can you do about children needing to stay home? If you're in the middle class, you were likely an over-worked parent already, and you are now tasked with homeschooling. I see remote-schooling laments on social media frequently, and there is a healthy dose of truth in them. No individual parent, of course, is responsible for any of this; it could even be argued that policy decisions made this outcome inevitable. What I *am* saying is that if we had been prepared to be prepared, things might have gone differently. And we all have a role in being prepared to be prepared in the future by ridding ourselves of problematic illusions about death, dying, and disease, and being more willing to "step up."

———

I said before, in **Lesson 6**, that there is no zero-risk situation; we simply choose the risks we take. And we must take risks, because we must be able to have some sort of society to return to once the COVID-19 pandemic is behind us. As humans participating in a society, whether we like it or not, we have a symbiotic relationship with economies. But it's important to remember that

LESSON 24:
The fallout already existed—
it was just more convenient to ignore.

On the other hand, just as firmly as I believe schools are a necessary social and cognitive learning space for children, I equally as firmly believe we as a country—parents and nonparents alike—need to consider the role public schools have come to play in our lives. One of the biggest concerns across America as grade schools contemplated shutdowns was what some kids were going to eat. Hundreds of thousands of children in America depend upon free breakfasts and lunches at schools. In fact, many schools send qualifying children home with food each weekend, to make sure they have meals when they're *not* at school. And while I could hypothetically imagine scenarios in which this is unavoidably the only safe way for many children to have food, in most cases, I think the problem is much simpler: the child's family is food insecure. I'm glad schools come to the rescue for these children, of course. But I think the COVID-19 shutdowns, particularly where our biggest social concern about closing schools was that it would leave many children hungry, has opened an important question for us in the United States, one we can potentially use, should we choose to, as a spark for growth and progress. Why are educational institutions our most certain, most foolproof means of making sure our own citizens don't go hungry? Couldn't we—*shouldn't we*—find a better way to feed our nation's children?

My friend Caitlin Tumlinson, a teacher, gave me an interesting example of the education system's problems being highlighted by the novel coronavirus. To add to the example of concrete resource scarcity, consider this: in many cases, even when computers are sent home to allow students to do their online schooling, in Caitlin's district and, undoubtedly, many others around the country, students are bussed *right back in* to use the school's internet![4] Here again, the image of students sitting yards apart from one another in empty school cafeterias doing their *fully remote learning from inside the school* because they don't have internet at home should make us pause. Why aren't we yet treating the internet like a public good that everyone needs?

---

4   Caitlin Tumlinson, MS NBCT, personal communication.

On a similar note, as many other overworked parents-turned-homeschool-teachers can attest, I think our nation should consider whether or not we have used free public schooling as a stand-in for daycare. In considering questions like this, my first move is to compare my country's experiences and practices with those around the world. It's hard to deny that the very existence of a system that houses children for nine hours a day is going to preclude parents hiring daily care for their children—regardless of what nation we examine. This problem seems to exist worldwide, simply because pretty much worldwide, we expect our children to be in school, and no alternatives have been required before now.

Americans have somehow turned one of life's greatest joys—that of watching our children grow up—into an economic burden that cripples families who can just barely afford it, and has simultaneously made the people who should be guiding and educating our children the ones responsible for their nutrition, daycare, and access to basic functional resources. This serves neither teachers nor our children. My husband is a teacher, so believe me when I say that I respect the fact that they do all these things. But should they *have* to? How much better could they be at teaching if they weren't also expected to be truancy police, nutrition providers, and babysitters, all the while trying to cram algebra down the next generation's throats? So, while we need schools just like we need economies, we ought to be very carefully examining what we've made of our education system. Isn't the ridiculous situation of remote-but-not-remote education a crystal-clear illustration that something wrong is woven into the very fabric of our social systems? Examining exactly *what* was disrupted in our lives when schooling was paused can reveal incredibly important places where we need to improve these systems. Parents, when they can, are still paying daycares to watch their school-age children and monitor their digital school progress. Why have we built a society with no affordable childcare options for parents when emergencies do arise, one where basic goods for living must be provided by the places that are supposed to simply educate our children?

Lest you think this professor is going to let higher education off the hook, I'm going to say something I'm very nervous to put on paper: I believe that the system of higher education in America has become one that has also commodified the bodies of our college-age citizens—and in this case, the colleges themselves become the participants in a bidding war to get high school seniors to choose them over other schools. I'm nervous to say this, because I think that as far as possible, my current workplace is in many ways an exception to these rules, and I don't want to be accused of either disloyalty or insincerity. Never have I seen a school more committed to ethical practices in regard to their students, faculty, and staff than Whitworth University; it is a testament to their safe and innovative practices for in-person return that Whitworth never had more than twenty-eight cases of COVID-19 at one time among the entire faculty, staff, and student population.[5] I think most institutions should take a moment and learn from how Whitworth implemented its return to campus, and I'm reluctant to say anything that could be misconstrued as having drawn this critique in any practical way from what I've witnessed there. But this is not a problem of any individual institution; it's a problem with the system as a whole, and universities have had to play the game or shut down. When old, wealthy universities like Brown publicly announce that many universities can't afford *not* to return to in-person schooling after the spring 2020 shutdown (which in my humble opinion may indicate that Brown itself also believes it cannot afford it), you can hardly imagine that smaller schools have the slightest chance of survival without students returning to campus. For one thing, students are simply not going to pay the current tuition rates in America—an average of $41,411 at private colleges and

---

5 Randy Michaelis, PhD, personal communication.

anywhere from $11,171 to $26,809 for state universities, depending on residency—to attend online school.[6] They will instead attend community colleges. But private and large four-year public schools have gotten into a "Business Model of Education," as historian and academic Bret Devereaux notes.[7] By this he means that universities increasingly attempt to run themselves like businesses, where students are seen as customers. And because, as he notes, "only a handful of nationally known big schools can compete on raw prestige," the vast majority of schools must compete on the amenities and lifestyle they can offer students. These very amenities are, of course, what has driven college tuition sky high in recent years but also what has attracted those very students.

Yes, I bristle a bit when I hear the beer pong parties in my neighborhood, and I do my part to break them up. There's no doubt in my mind that they could easily spread COVID-19. But I also bristle at the very notion that universities across the nation have persuaded—upon pain of institutional death if they fail—tens of thousands of young adults to return to school, and then been angry, shocked, or surprised when these young adults . . . well, behaved like young adults. As I suggested in the opening to this chapter, college kids are more or less *supposed* to behave the way they do. What I've seen around me is college-age students turned into dollar signs and then criticized nationwide for doing what any reasonable person could have expected them to do. It's hard for me to even blame the large state schools that I think had far less justification in returning students to campus: the system of higher education, as it currently exists, means that almost

---

6　Farran Powell and Emma Kerr, "What You Need to Know about College Tuition Costs," *U.S. News & World Report*, September 17, 2020, www.usnews.com/education/best-colleges/paying-for-college/articles/what-you-need-to-know-about-college-tuition-costs.

7　Bret Devereaux, Twitter post, August 18, 2020, https://twitter.com/BretDevereaux/.

every university across the country subsists paycheck to paycheck. Many truly would go out of business—and that's a term I use intentionally here—if an additional semester of school were fully digital. What is the ethical choice when a total institutional shutdown could mean the loss of thousands of jobs internally, and even more in cities with businesses and industries built around college students? What about the lived lives of people who don't die but find difficulty putting food on the table now that they're unemployed? Or people who can't get new work because their city has become a ghost town? In my opinion these are real and valuable concerns as well, and while it may seem simple to say we should protect biological life at any cost, a statement like that far too easily sidesteps looking in the face of exactly what that cost is. At the same time, it seems to me that we are commodifying the bodies of all our youth—the very young at the many dollars per hour of care that parents need to cough up, and our young adults at the price of their education. In many other countries, all of these services—daycare, parental leave, and higher education—are subsidized by the government, and capitalism still chugs on. Here in the United States, we seem to be more inclined to put prices on people's heads, a choice that predictably penalizes already marginalized groups. As I said in **Lesson 5**, it is absolutely possible to maintain a capitalist economy while also serving the needs of a country's citizens.

If the 1918 influenza pandemic taught us one thing, it was that we couldn't depend upon standard wisdom to predict who was going to get sick, or who was going to be the most vulnerable to a disease. Making assumptions about the limits of who a disease will harm only allows time for the disease to call our bluff as it spreads. Whether we're thinking of the impact from the disease itself or if we consider broader social and cultural impacts, pandemic disease by its very nature leaves no one untouched. Instead, it creates an unacknowledged Lost Generation—much like that of 1918—who fall through the cracks, whose lives and troubles impact the world for generations, as they work, form relationships, and parent. The inverse is equally true: assuming a disease will impact *only some* groups is, in my thinking, a weakness that pathogens will exploit readily, and the following chapters cover this subject in depth.

9

THE GREAT SOCIAL LEVELER

How STDs Called Privilege's Bluff
(and How the New Coronavirus
Will Call Ours, Too)

1885 *and* 1985

Portsmouth, UK
January 1, 1873

Julia Clark contemplated her bowl of soup. She looked across the table at Laura, who was voraciously slurping hers down, and then looked back to her own bowl, weighing her hunger against her anger. She was pretty hungry, but *boy* was she angry. Throwing her shoulders back and situating herself a little taller in her seat, she glanced furtively at the other women eating in the mess hall with her. She knew many of them were angry, too, and those who weren't avowedly angry were desperate. She knew from experience that desperation made people bold. Bold enough to do the unladylike, the unthinkable . . .

She looked around the room once more, this time toward the head matron, and she felt her resolve strengthen. Leading a crew of like-minded, angry, and desperate women in a quasi-violent revolution *might* end with her own solitary punishment—*I might even be convicted of assault!* she thought to herself. *But it could also end in change* . . . Still, she was nervous.

She bit her lower lip and took a deep breath. Then she grabbed her soup bowl and hurled it at the head matron's skull. Her eyes lit up as she saw the air immediately filled with flying soup. Chaos had been unleashed.

In 1873, a food fight (known as the "soup riot") in a hospital dining room symbolized decades of building tensions.[1] What makes an otherwise seemingly random, juvenile incident relevant? The patients, mostly female, were prisoners. Their crime? Having syphilis. Because of this, they had been locked away in specialized hospitals (called Lock Hospitals) for what must have felt like arbitrary durations, and in this particular instance, they'd had enough. The context leading up to this moment in disease history is important, because it teaches us that

Lesson 25: Not-obvious plague is . . . not obvious.

Lesson 26: What's in a name? Everything.

Lesson 27: Disease language affects disease spread.

Before explaining what led up to the funny-but-serious soup riot, however, it will be helpful to preface this explanation with another example.

---

1   I'm forever grateful to Judith Walkowitz's amazing book *Prostitution and Victorian Society: Women, Class, and the State* (Cambridge, UK: Cambridge University Press, 1980) for this fascinating anecdote, which can be found on page 215.

I imagine it like this. Catherine, Marchioness of Camden (or wherever; it doesn't really matter, I made her up), came down to breakfast at half past nine, as she had every morning of her ten-year marriage. The scones and kedgeree were placed at her end of the table for her to serve her husband, per her standing request. To have been married for a decade, to dine together each morning to this day, and for Catherine to demurely serve her husband his scone lightly basted with clotted cream with her own hands—these were signs of a happy marriage in British high society in the 1880s. Most couples didn't regularly eat together, and for a rich woman with a title to serve her husband his food was considered a loving gesture to which few wives of such status condescended.

But this morning something changed. Catherine was accustomed to reading the newspaper while she waited for her husband to join her, as she had always been the earlier riser. Perhaps it wasn't exactly ladylike to read the science and engineering sections in the paper with zeal, but she loved the information they held. It was a delightfully simple way of apprising herself of the most recent goings-on without wasting her entire morning. She usually found the industrial announcements in the section rather boring, but it did make her a lively conversant at parties. She arched an eyebrow at what she read today, though: "*tubercule . . . characterized and caused by a bacillus . . . the expectorations from the lungs of consumptives are full of these bacilli . . . it is extremely dangerous to inhale air in which this contagious dust may have mingled.*"[2] Her eyes flashed over the words, skipping the details but gathering the significance. Could consumption itself (that's what the Victorians called TB) be *contagious*? She considered this novel possibility as she poured the tea.

---

2   These words are taken from an actual report of Robert Koch's famous discovery: *London Evening Standard*, May 1, 1882, 7.

A slight cough announced Henry's entrance into the room, and she glanced up and deftly filled another teacup for him. He coughed again and her arm hitched slightly, spilling steaming tea drops on the dark wood of the table. She watched him carefully as he seated himself, and she kept watching him as she daintily carried his teacup and scone toward him. Her own habitual cough occasionally echoed his. Henry had always had a cough since long before they were married—hay fever, his family had always said—but her own she'd blamed on the drafty rooms in the east wing, where her apartments were.

Now back at her own seat, she studied Henry from across the table. *Could he have . . . possibly . . . infected her?* The teacup made a hollow sound as it clattered on the floor, its delicate china pattern scattered into a million incoherent parts that could never be pieced together again.

Which brings us to

LESSON 25:
Not-obvious plague is . . . not obvious.
(aka The Mini-Chapter: The TB Shuffle)

Susan Sontag has likened tuberculosis in the nineteenth century to cancer in our day: both are poorly understood, and therefore explanations of causes and cures shift and mold according to society's unconscious biases and beliefs (hey there, **SSDC**! Ahem, **Lesson 20**). Frankly, I could devote an entire chapter to TB and what it could teach us, but because I think most of its lessons are similar to those of many venereal diseases— for reasons that will become clear shortly—instead I've opted to include it simply as a lengthy subpoint in this chapter on syphilis and HIV.

TB absolutely befuddled Victorian society. Long after the heyday of germ theory took the world by storm, in fact long after the TB microbe was identified by Robert Koch in 1882, people *still* debated whether or not TB was contagious. *How is this so*, you might be asking? *The evidence was right there, under the microscope! No one questioned the various other disease microbes discovered this way!* After all, we've had nearly two whole chapters explaining the vast problems associated with *overly eager* acceptance of germ theory's findings. Let's try explanation by way of video game, shall we?

In *Plague Inc.*, the user plays as a microbe attempting to destroy all of humanity. It's morbid, I know, but I use it in my medical humanities classes to get students thinking about digital design surrounding health topics. It's truly a pretty well-designed game. When you play it enough, you quickly learn that the subtle diseases are the most effective. What defines a "subtle" pathogen? Two things, generally, in the game (and in life): diseases with slow incubation periods, and diseases that don't make people very sick at first—in other words, diseases that take a long time to kill their hosts. And, indeed, history bears out the truth of this strategy.

I've mentioned this before, when discussing the "birth" of the concept of contagion: some diseases were known to be contagious *long before* germ theory, generally because they were simply visually noticeable, as was their quick spread. If you run into someone who has smallpox sores all over their body and you touch them, and then you get smallpox sores all over your body just a few days later, contagion is simply the logical answer. The equation here is simple:

Visible markings unique to a specific disease
+ quick incubation time
_____

obvious linear connection between points
of contact.

This was accepted even before germ theory existed. The opposite is also true, and possibly even more important (it is certainly more relevant to COVID-19).

Long incubation time
+ a disease with few obvious visual markers

---

people will not automatically realize
said disease is contagious.

Even in our scientifically and technologically advanced age, quantitative research can only begin in earnest when a suspicion of a connection—often noticed *qualitatively*—exists in the first place. In the case of tuberculosis, skepticism over its contagious nature remained prevalent long past the discovery of its microbe. Tuberculosis is a funny disease; to the Victorians, it seemed wily, and it was poorly understood. The disease was rampant in nineteenth-century Britain—it's thought that up to 25 percent of the entire English population in 1815 had the disease, and that it was responsible for 30 percent of English deaths by 1830.[3] Yet TB is actually a pretty weak pathogen. Only about 33 percent of people exposed to it will actually contract the disease itself—it predominantly affects immunocompromised people.[4] Of this percentage, only a further 10 percent will actually ever *show symptoms* of active infection. For the rest of the folks who actually contract the disease, it will remain latent in their system indefinitely. To make the disease's trajectory more confusing, *if* a person develops an active infection (and remember, this may never happen even in those who have technically contracted the disease), it may be years—maybe even a decade—until it appears. In fact, it was *because* TB was a fairly weak pathogen that it could *become* the global threat that it was (and remains today). It wasn't

---

3 Carol Dyer, *Tuberculosis: Biographies of Disease* (Santa Barbara, CA: Greenwood, 2010), 36.

4 Issar Smith, "*Mycobacterium tuberculosis* Pathogenesis and Molecular Determinants of Virulence," *Clinical Microbiology Review* 16 (2003): 493–96.

as though you could eyeball Joe from down the block and have any certainty that his cough caused your cough ten years later. And even *then* you could live for years and years with nothing but a cough and some complexion changes. TB might easily mimic a simple cough or cold for some time in a patient. TB moved slowly, and it killed slowly . . . and subtly. Though it did have certain recognizable signs (like a cough), such symptoms could mean any number of things, as we of course know from the era of COVID-19, when seasonal allergies can instill panic in any one of us.

What's more, many of the symptoms of TB seemed almost gentle, pretty even. Historian Carolyn Day has written an entire book on the consumptive chic (also the title of the book), in which she tracks a variety of fashion trends from the late eighteenth and early nineteenth centuries that tried to mimic the "look" of someone with TB. There were whitening powders that could give people a tubercular pallor, rouges to give the feverish, flushed look to the cheeks, and even gowns designed to give the stooped-shoulder look of patients with TB. It might seem odd to call a disease "gentle," especially a fatal one like TB, but remember how absolutely chock full of disease the world was at this time, many of them nasty suckers that we don't really see much anymore in the new millennium. Compared to diseases like cholera, which caused people to eject their insides out into the room around them, or puerperal fever, which turned women's insides black (such features were observed during autopsies), the pale complexion and rosy cheeks of tuberculosis could indeed seem rather slow and gentle. And lest you curl your lip at the "tubercular chic" fashion trends of the early 1800s, let me remind you of the "heroin chic" trend that pervaded catwalks in the early 1990s. As Sontag says, when we don't know what to make of a disease, we tend to bend it to whatever purposes we need it to serve. The less clear a disease's epidemiology is, the more of a blank slate or an inkblot test it becomes for us, saying much more about us than it does the pathogen. As famous TB researchers Rene and Jean Dubos explain, "Diseases manifest multiple personalities . . . [and] the various moods which they display . . . reflect the dominant aspect of the relationship between the disease process and the life of many in society."[5] All of these factors meant that as late as 1912, famous statistician (and eugenicist—boo, hiss) Karl Pearson could write an *entire book* debating the contagiousness of tuberculosis.[6] The parallel here to COVID-19 is obvious, I hope.

Subtle, slow diseases are confusing to the naked eye and to our anecdotal experience of the world, making their spread harder to see for ourselves (more on this in the next lessons and subsequent chapter). This makes public buy-in to containment an uphill battle already (recall **Lessons 12 and 19**: we need belief and buy-in). Adding to the difficulties of buy-in, however, is that when a society is confused about a disease, it becomes that blank slate I mentioned earlier, capable of containing all of society's biases and prejudices. More often than not, the disease *itself* becomes stigmatized. Think of leprosy, for instance. Perhaps more than any other historic disease, leprosy is most familiar to laypeople (meaning you folks who don't spend your every waking moment thinking about disease and bodies like me). Why? Because the Bible, a book seemingly about everything *but* leprosy, is curiously *full* of decrees about how to handle the disease. Leprosy is actually caused by a pathogen very similar in biochemical structure to TB, and

---

5   Rene Dubos and Jean Dubos, *The White Plague: Tuberculosis, Man, and Society* (New Brunswick, NJ: Rutgers University Press, 1987), 3, quoted in Nixon, *Kept from All Contagion*, 101.

6   Back in my statistician days, I almost named my beloved dog, subject of my "death article" for *YES!* magazine, Pearson, after Karl Pearson. This was before I knew his Victorian history—I knew him only as the creator of the majestic Pearson Product Moment Correlation Coefficient. It would only be later that I would learn of his history as a *person*—a bad one, at that. I'm so glad I named the dog Oberon, after the king of the fairies, instead.

although it has obvious visible markers, leprosy's spread was confusing to many societies. People thought that displaying symptoms of leprosy perhaps meant you'd come into contact with something unclean or sacrilegious. Hence, it became its own taboo, so deeply ingrained in our cultural understanding that even thousands of years later, we know what the disease is.

People will always exploit disease as a way to fuel prejudices they already have. This is even more true regarding venereal diseases, simply by virtue of their being "sexually transmitted diseases." In the 1860s (remember the food fight?), syphilis was seen as evidence of sexual vice and was readily construed as the collective sin of sex workers alone in a male-dominated society. In other words, men, the usual customers of sex workers, were "off the hook," so to speak—at least in the collective imagination. Early-stage syphilis is marked by small lesions on the skin that come and go, and so sufferers and physicians alike often thought of it as a disease that cured itself, much like we might think about a cold sore (although we benefit from modern microbiology, which teaches us that the *disease* is still there, even if its symptoms aren't). Recall that we're talking about the same era as Semmelweis here, so disease concepts in general were much more flexible, and syphilis, as notorious as it is culturally, can in fact be a very subtle creature in the body. Based on clinical signs alone—which is all society had at the time—it was easy enough to believe that the disease resolved itself. Its telltale genital lesions wax and wane across the course of the disease, and although syphilis does eventually ramp up and kill, this can occur years after the fact. "Chaste" Victorian men believed only sex workers spread the disease—or at least that controlling their bodies would fully control the spread of syphilis, which is akin to saying the same thing—and a series of laws called the Contagious Disease Acts were passed to control the bodies of sex workers. According to these laws, any woman suspected of being a sex worker could be detained by police and subjected to forcible speculum examination to determine if she had signs of syphilis.

Spoiler alert: Victorian prudery meant a lot of men were not so great at distinguishing symptoms of syphilis from ordinary female bodily functions, and so a *lot* of women were at risk of being deemed syphilitic. If such a diagnosis was made, the woman was sent to detainment in a Lock Hospital until she improved.

Spoiler alert #2: Penicillin didn't exist yet, so people didn't really get better. Eventually, a doctor might declare an inmate past the infectious stage of the disease (according to contemporary medical beliefs), but if a woman happened to have lesions that weren't resolving or normal vaginal discharge completely unrelated to syphilis that lingered because it was *normal,* she could be subject to a sentence of up to nine months.

Take a moment and imagine that. Imagine living a life where you could be swept off the street, forced to undergo what amounts to rape by instrument, and then jailed for up to nine months, possibly because you may or may not have had syphilis, and possibly because you may or may not have been a sex worker (although being a sex worker justifies none of the above, anyway).

What's that, you say? Yes, this law threatened *all women* because of the difficulty of identifying sex workers. Shockingly, they look just like the rest of us humans (if you don't read that statement as dripping with sarcasm, then you might be reading the wrong book). Were you a woman out after dark without a chaperone? You were at risk of being deemed a sex worker and forced to undergo examination and possible detention. Were you a woman out after dark *with* a chaperone, but one that people didn't recognize? He might have been a client, and you, too, were at risk of being deemed a sex worker, and thus abused and jailed. The laws were so horrific that even Victorians themselves—

hardly known for a status quo that championed women's rights—were horrified by them, and the laws were repealed in 1886. Public outrage definitely fueled the repeal efforts, but so did something else: the development of macroscopic evidence that supported by-then accepted microbiological theories about disease's spread. For some time, it was possible to believe that "chaste" Victorian men who happened to consort with sex workers could be somehow saved from the disease if the sex workers' bodies were controlled strictly enough. That is, until their "good" and "chaste" Victorian wives—who were *not* consorting with sex workers—began giving birth to babies with congenital syphilis, both mother and child having been infected by a philandering husband. Babies with congenital syphilis were very distinctive looking, and many Victorians saw the spike in congenital syphilis as its own plague, a reaper coming to claim its due from a society that thought its systemic abuse and blaming of the marginalized could continue with impunity. HIV, which often (though not always) has a long latency period that can often be relatively asymptomatic, functioned in much the same way in the 1980s. Like leprosy and TB, these diseases work in mysterious ways that are often not visible to human observation in the short term. But because syphilis and HIV are venereal diseases, their use as vehicles to fuel existing biases against marginalized populations is even greater, because

LESSON 26:
What's in a name? Everything.

What makes a sexually transmitted disease a sexually transmitted disease? The answer probably seems obvious—it's even built into the designator of "sexually transmitted disease." And that's my point. As I mentioned in the previous lesson, at least in Western society, the very label of something as sexually transmitted is by definition stigmatized because sex itself has become a taboo. This changes the algebra quite a bit. Remember:

> Long incubation time
> + a disease with few obvious visual markers
>
> ---
>
> people will not automatically realize said disease is contagious and will therefore interpret the disease however suits their needs/existing belief systems, possibly building taboos around it.

Now, add to this equation:

> Knowledge/belief that a disease is acquired through an already taboo act (here, sex)
> + long incubation time
> + a disease with few obvious visual markers
>
> ---
>
> a predetermined stigmatizing view of anyone who has said disease.

And *presto!* You have a recipe that tends to greatly disadvantage already marginalized populations. It's almost as if this epidemiological system was *made* to target people who are already treated as "less than" by our society. But hark! What's that I hear? Is it the siren song of the socio-scientific discursive cycle calling to us? (If you need a refresher, flip back to **Lesson 20**, because what I'm about to say is important.) If my medical humanities training has taught me anything—and hopefully if this book has taught you anything—it's that when a scientific "fact" seems a little too consistently convenient for a group in power, we need to explore how this fact has been made, to make sure that it's actually scientific fact (see **Lesson 18**) rather than simply a reflection of our own cultural biases (**Lesson 25**). That's the tricky thing about being a medical humanist: convincing people that we medical humanities scholars are not in the business of "debunking" science. Rather, we hope to make *better* science by exposing the ways that science is the product of (drumroll, please, for Steven Shapin), *People with Bodies, Situated in Time, Space, Culture, and Society, and Struggling for Credibility and Authority.* If we are unwilling to explore all the ways science could in fact be conveniently replicating what we want to believe in the world (and yes, for all its numbers and statistics meant to solidify its objectivity, it certainly can be inadvertently doing just that), then we *will* be subject to accidental biases infecting our science, and we will exist in a world with very problematic beliefs. Consider the implicit bias of a series of Victorian laws that acted as though sex workers were the sole "conduit of infection to respectable society."[7] While they may have known realistically that disease spread through sex workers' clients as well, the laws nevertheless represented a cultural fantasy (a zeitgeist, if you will, as per **Lesson 24**) that somehow the disease could be willed to stay only in certain bodies. It's all well and good to chuckle at "silly" Victorian beliefs, but don't we to this day continue to construe HIV to be mostly a problem of the homosexual population? For these reasons, humor me as I ask you again: What makes a disease "sexually transmitted"?

———

Let's try out some different answers to this question and see if they hold water.

Possible Answer 1: An STD is a disease transmitted by sex.

---

7   Walkowitz, *Prostitution and Victorian Society*, 4.

Again, this seems obvious. But what about a cold contracted by breathing near someone during sex? We don't call that an STD. Of course not, you might say, because a cold can be contracted many *other* ways than through sex. Which leads us to:

Possible Answer 2: An STD is a disease transmitted through sexual fluids.

Here we've ruled out colds and diseases that could be contracted through sex but whose primary mechanism has nothing to do with sex. So where do we stand with a disease like Ebola? Studies in 2014 showed that the Ebola virus was indeed carried through seminal fluid. Well, says the devil's advocate in us, like the common cold, Ebola *can* be contracted through sex, but is also contracted through other means. Yet our answers are getting weaker, because Ebola can nevertheless be transmitted *specifically* through sexual fluids. Okay, let's try this one on for size:

Possible Answer 3: An STD is a disease transmitted *primarily* through sexual fluids, rather than other means.

But what about HIV? Unless you've done a lot of research on HIV, you might be surprised that I've introduced HIV as a counterpoint to this argument. I can't speak for everyone, of course, but in my experience, as I was taught about HIV via videos shown in my public-school classrooms, I was at the same time taught that HIV was a disease transmitted by sex and that safe sex was the answer. In fact, HIV's most viable means of contagious spread is through blood, just like Ebola. In many regards, we could just as easily consider HIV more akin to simply a bloodborne pathogen than specifically a disease of sexual activity. Anal sex does increase the risk of HIV, but only because it has a tendency to tear sensitive tissue and expose blood vessels.

So, I ask you again: What makes an STD an STD? English professor Lucinda Cole has written and spoken about the taboos of eating carrion (which, surprisingly, have implications for the next chapter on

Ebola and its relationship to COVID-19). One of Cole's major points regarding societies that have taboos around eating carrion *and* for how humans classify animals as hunters or scavengers was a similar question that concerned the following: How long must something be dead for it to be considered carrion? A minute? An hour? When exactly does fresh meat turn into something we revile as unclean? How long must it sit, dead, before it converts in our minds to something it hadn't been before? Cole's examples are incredibly important for thinking through the difficult question I've posed here. I say *difficult* because I'm asking you to reconsider a zeitgeist (**Lesson 21**), and it is amazingly hard work to think outside the given "facts" of our world.

Just how important must sex be to the transmission of a disease to declare it "sexually transmitted"? Must 90 percent of the transmissions be through sex? Seventy-five percent of them? Fifty-one percent? Just what titration of infectious particles must be found in semen or vaginal fluids alone, rather than in the blood, for a disease to qualify as one sort of pathogen or the other? What kinds of sex matter in defining a disease as an STD? Though it may be difficult to think outside the rules we've been given about how to code these diseases, doing so is incredibly important work, because as the so-called good Victorian mothers discovered as they birthed babies with congenital syphilis,

LESSON 27:
Disease language affects disease spread.

This is one of the toughest lessons of this book, and it's kind of hard to swallow: our social biases are germs' secret weapon. Our infighting—even our unconscious judgments—allow them to gain a foothold of infection in humanity. It's the open door inviting them in, while we're expecting them to knock. For example, the longer Victorian society thought syphilis, a sexually transmitted disease, would logically only affect those most engaged in sex work, the more it had a chance to spread throughout Victorian society while everyone looked the other way at the red herring of their own making.

So, it makes sense that the longer heteronormative society coded HIV as a disease of homosexual vice, which to them justified ignoring this public health crisis, the more the virus was able to spread. It used our social prejudices against us to spread into more and more sectors of the population. Yes, the first publicized outbreaks in America happened in gay communities, but how much of that had to do with our ability to demarcate and recognize these groups as "different" to begin with? To put it another way, the first thing any epidemiologist or contact tracer is going to do when a new infectious disease appears is to look for similarities between the infected and *differences* between the infected and the uninfected. These differences are observed with subjective human reason—they do not exist in the atmosphere, waiting for us to pluck them, preformed, from some Tree of Knowledge. So, the differences we look for are going to be the differences we have already created ourselves as a society (such as differences in sexual orientation or practice). Which means (and buckle up for this next one): *any* difference we observe in *social* practices is a difference we have created.

It isn't hard to imagine sexual orientation difference—something that unfortunately decidedly marks difference in our society—as being meaningless in another culture, say, on another planet. I could readily see a populace that simply defined sexual activity as occurring between humans, making no distinction regarding gender. In fact, scholars of the Victorian era like Linda Dowling have gone so far as to suggest that our binary view of sexuality—which prevailed and arguably still prevails—is something also developed more recently. She suggests that such a binary view of sexuality didn't even exist in the Victorian era, a time period that is so easy for us to imagine as backward.

The point here is that we can only see lifestyle differences as they appear to be different or unusual or meaningful to us, and that is entirely subject to how we see the world around us to begin with. It's something of a self-fulfilling prophecy that in a society that already sees homosexuality as "different" (and this was even more so in the 1980s than it is today), when we notice a disease occur in that population, their "different" status (here, homosexuality) is going to be (problematically) the starting point for our disease investigation. As Steven Epstein puts it in *Impure Science*, "the difficulty is that the isolation of 'difference' presupposes a common understanding of what constitutes the 'background' against which this difference stands out. In this sense, epidemiology is inevitably a 'normalizing' science, employing—and reinforcing—unexamined notions of normality to measure and classify deviations from the norm."[8]

From there, when you consider how our society stigmatizes homosexuality to begin with, it's all too easy to see that "scientific" conclusions may have too readily identified homosexual behavior as the cause of HIV, at the expense of data that demonstrates needle users, blood transfusion recipients, and heterosexual couples often fall victim to the disease as well. In fact, in the 1980s, the CDC task force on the new disease noted that only 8 percent of observed cases occurred in homosexuals, and at least one of those cases was a female.[9] Indeed, as Epstein notes, "if gay men were perceived as *plausible* victims of a medical syndrome, it was in part because in the medical literature their sexualized lifestyle was already depicted as medically problematic."[10] This epidemiological misstep then makes it far too easy to miss cases, allowing the disease to spread like wildfire while we point fingers at

---

8 Steven Epstein, *Impure Science: AIDS, Activism, and the Politics of Knowledge* (Berkeley: University of California Press, 1996), 49.

9 Ibid., 47.

10 Ibid., 50.

those we'd most like to blame to begin with. This is the socio-scientific discursive cycle at work (**Lesson 20**).

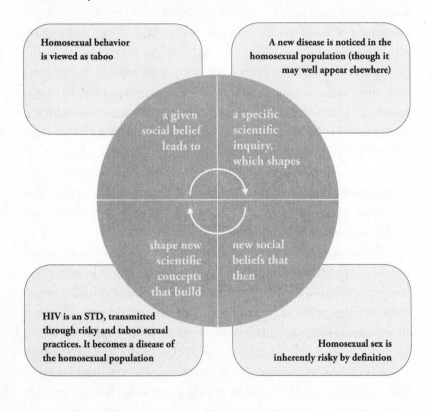

The drag queen's bouffant was *impeccable*, and her plum purple power suit set it off perfectly. Against the background music of a *killer* drumbeat and the backdrop of a golden chandelier, her confidence was calming even to the viewer as she said matter-of-factly, "For Kings, this Queen, and you royals in between," with a flashy flip of her wrist.[11] Lest you think this is a problem relegated to the 1980s, I've seen the

11   "Descovy for PrEP Commercial," www.youtube.com/watch?v=nhsF7Csninw.

problematic bias of HIV as a disease of the homosexual population perpetuated as late as January 2020, even in spaces meant to empower them. This particular instance was in a commercial for Descovy, a proactive medication meant to lower the risk of HIV contraction during sex. However, only cisgender men and trans women are represented in the commercial. One very twitterpated couple even breaks the fourth wall, explaining: "Descovy has not been studied in people assigned female at birth." Here is an even more blatant demonstration of the SSDC at work. In this case, we have essentially the second cycle, facilitated by the early biases in the diagram above. First, we begin from the bottom left point on the diagram. The final step on the above cycle now becomes our beginning sociological belief—our new starting point. From here, existing social beliefs have led a pharmaceutical company to only deem drug safety studies necessary or valuable to conduct in men. Because of this, the medicine can only legally be marketed to men in commercials like this. Such media portrayals further strengthen a cultural attitude that portrays HIV as a disease of homosexual men, and this likely continues to hinder scientific inquiries about other impacted populations.

The first iteration of the SSDC in regard to HIV (shown above) is well documented as the prevailing zeitgeist in the 1980s, which greatly delayed the development of treatments for HIV. It was all too easy for an already prejudiced society to ignore a disease they thought they were somehow safe from (more on this in the next chapter), but this quite literal ignorance continues to impact the way we construct science, medicine, and social beliefs today. I personally think it's incredibly dangerous to perpetuate the idea that HIV is prevalent in only one portion of our society. This only allows HIV a foothold from which to grow, while we bury our heads in the sand and pretend that some of us are somehow exempt from a virus that can infect all humans. Typically, social histories of HIV recount that when the hemophiliac population began to test positive for HIV, the focus shifted to exploring bloodborne pathogen etiologies. Yet isn't it simultaneously true that society became motivated to further explore causal explanations *because* the disease had now spread to a community they imagined as "innocent" and undeserving of infectious disease? To return to TB, most scientists consider the disease a "conditional" one, so weak it only causes disease in humans in the context of certain environmental factors such as malnutrition or overcrowding.[12] Here again, we see a disease that society all too readily ignored in Victorian England because it affected the working poor, and one that we continue to ignore today because it affects the Third World—globally, COVID-19 killed 1.8 million people in 2020; TB kills around 1.4 million *every year*. By the mid-nineteenth century, however, it was time to pay the piper. Victorian upper-class disregard for the living conditions of the poor came back to haunt them, as it had in fact allowed for tuberculosis's rampant spread among all parts of the country.

It took far too long for HIV drugs to be developed because, among other things, it really seemed like the Reagan administration didn't care about diseases that affected an "othered" group like homosexuals. How many more medicines like Descovy might we have for *everyone* if we stopped construing it as a disease of homosexual men? Why, even now, is America and the West so fixated on "the AIDS crisis in Africa" while the publicity about our own HIV patients has lost momentum? My friend Sarah McDonald put it best while we were sitting at my table discussing this book one morning as I prepared for a day of writing. Her profound words have haunted me ever since: "White saviorism has claimed the problem of AIDS in Africa but failed in America because here it was mostly projected onto the LGBTQ population.

---

12 Chai Qiyao, Yong Zhang, and Cui Hua Liu, "*Mycobacterium tuberculosis*: An Adaptable Pathogen Associated with Multiple Human Diseases," *Frontiers in Cellular and Infection Microbiology* 8 (2018).

White saviorism doesn't have a place for the LGBTQ population, so it ignores them."[13]

I think she's spot-on. And the problem—aside from bigotry and neocolonialism—is that when we "don't have a place" for problems of groups we see as "Other" in our world, disease-causing germs have already won. You see, they don't care how we label each other, or who we make a place for at the table. Their only directive is to spread. And when we deny a place at the table for those we deem "Other," pathogens help themselves to seconds.

---

13 Sarah McDonald, personal communication.

10

THE HOT ZONE

How One Author Launched an Ebola Fear Campaign That Still Hinders Pandemic Containment Today

1994

You would not have been able to ignore the man who was getting sick. . . . He is holding an airsickness bag over his mouth. He coughs a deep cough and regurgitates something into the bag. The bag swells up. . . . The connective tissue in his face is dissolving, and his face appears to hang off from the underlying bone, as if the face is detaching itself from the skull. He opens his mouth and gasps into the bag, and the vomiting goes on endlessly. It will not stop.[1]

---

1 Richard Preston, *The Hot Zone* (New York: Anchor, 1993). This quote is also mentioned in Catherine Belling's essay "Dark Zones: The Ebola Body as a Configuration of Horror," which I will discuss at length later in this chapter.

This is not my own imagining. Instead, it is a description of Ebola virus that appeared in journalist Richard Preston's 1994 bestseller, *The Hot Zone: The Terrifying True Story of the Origins of the Ebola Virus*. The book spent over thirty weeks on *Publishers Weekly*'s bestseller list. Richard Preston says "You wouldn't have been able to ignore the man on the plane"—that is, the man vomiting up his guts because of Ebola virus. But we in fact *do* ignore so many of the ghastly diseases around the planet . . . as long as they're not happening to *us*. We tend to react to disease as natural in certain geographic places.[2] *Those* people over there just always have *that* disease. But when America finds eleven Ebola patients within its borders? Outbreak! The way we talk about disease isn't the only thing affected by our preexisting beliefs and biases. The way we *react* to disease is also dependent on what we already believe. The Ebola "outbreak" of 2014 demonstrates these facts, teaching us

Lesson 28:   What's in a name, part 2.

Lesson 29:   Xenophobia is fear, and fear facilitates denial.

Lesson 30:   Prejudice is a disease.

---

2   This argument derives from Claire Hooker, Chris Degeling, and Paul Mason's very compelling article "Dying a Natural Death: Ethics and Political Activism for Endemic Infectious Disease." Both this essay and Belling's (mentioned in the previous footnote) can be found in the essay collection *Endemic: Essays in Contagion Theory*, eds. Kari Nixon and Lorenzo Servitje (London: Palgrave, 2016). Both pieces will be addressed at length later in this chapter.

Monrovia, Liberia
September 15, 2014

Thomas shifted uneasily in the cab's front seat. Everyone was worried about Ebola just now, but here was Marthalene, his pregnant neighbor, who had just collapsed. He had rushed to her side without thinking. He was probably a little apprehensive, but he knew in his heart that the right thing to do was to help her. He put his arm around her and carried her to the taxi to the hospital. He rode with her and her family on the way there—they needed support. That's what good neighbors did. And he was a good neighbor.

It's interesting to me, and it will be of note in the lessons that follow, that we in the West call this disease Ebola—a name derived from a river in central Africa, though some people, perhaps more accurately, call it "caretaker's" disease. You see, Ebola is actually pretty hard to get, not that you'd know that from reading Preston's account. It takes direct contact with certain bodily fluids—usually blood, feces, or vomit—and for this material to then somehow get into your mouth or a cut, for you to get Ebola. In other words, it's not breathed in and is rarely transmitted through secondary surface contact. This means that transmission is something that most commonly happens through prolonged contact—physical contact—with someone who is already sick. In particular, it usually involves the sort of intimate contact involved in caring for a sick person—exposure to phlegm, blood, and the like. Yet for all Preston's other exaggerations, the Ebola virus does have a high mortality rate. The number varies depending on the specific strain of Ebola virus at play in any given outbreak, but the 2014 strain had a mortality rate of over 50 percent. Ironically, though (as **Lesson 25** demonstrates in some way), the faster a disease kills its hosts, the less time it has to spread. Overly virulent diseases can raze their own host supply. Violent symptoms may also be easier to identify in order to isolate patients. It's easy to see, then, how diseases like the novel coronavirus, with slow incubation periods and mild symptoms for most people, can sometimes be so surprisingly deadly for the population as a whole.

———

When he arrived in America, Thomas must have been so excited to see his partner and children, who had been living on the other side of an ocean for sixteen years.[3] I can only imagine the anticipation of that flight, and the drive from the airport to their apartment. And no, there wasn't a motion sickness bag full of vomit, nor flesh melting off his bones. In fact, when Thomas Eric Duncan first checked himself into Presbyterian Hospital in Dallas, Texas, on September 24, 2014, the doctors diagnosed him with a sinus infection and sent him home with some antibiotics. It was pretty anticlimactic at first, and it's quite possible that it was also steeped in systemic racial biases that may have very well cost Thomas his life. There are too many

---

3   Since his death, his partner, Louise Troh, has written a memoir about their life together, titled *My Spirit Took You In: The Romance That Sparked an Epidemic of Fear, A Memoir of the Life and Death of Thomas Eric Duncan, America's First Ebola Victim* (New York: Weinstein Books, 2015), excerpted in Louise Troh, "The Tragic Love Story behind America's First Ebola Victim," *Vanity Fair*, April 23, 2015, www.vanityfair.com/culture/2015/04/my-spirit-took-you-in-louise -troh-excerpt.

studies to count that demonstrate that Black people's pain and symptomatology are more likely to be ignored, dismissed, or discounted by those in the medical profession. To do justice to the topic would require another several books. Given this, it's interesting—and significant—that while Thomas Eric Duncan and a few others supposedly ushered an Ebola "outbreak" into the United States, which consisted of all of eleven patients, very few people died. Thomas did, though. So did a surgeon from Sierra Leone (who had permanent residency in America).

As I've said, Ebola isn't easy to catch. It is pretty dangerous once you have it, though. We don't exactly have antivirals in the same way we have antibiotics. They exist, of course, but there are fewer of them tailored to specific bugs, and they're incredibly hard on the body. They're reserved mostly for long-term viral load infections such as herpes, and even then only during flares, or HIV (the antiviral drug Tamiflu, which is used to treat influenza, is one notable exception). Like most viruses, treatment involves simply keeping the patient alive by hydrating them and providing oxygen or whatever else is needed by the body until the virus passes. But Thomas was sent home, at least initially, and likely until it was too late.

When all this happened, in 2014, I lived virtually within walking distance of Presbyterian Hospital. My husband once worked at the huge used bookstore—situated in a repurposed big-box sporting goods warehouse—that sat down the road from the apartment complex where Thomas's family lived, and where he came to stay with them. This small subsection of Dallas is known as Vickery Meadow, and it houses mostly low-income immigrants and refugees in a few blocks of different apartment complexes. The neighborhood itself is only 5.3 square miles in size, with most of its housing centered in a 2.8-square-mile section—in 2015, 27,047 people lived there, mostly in the apartments that characterize the area, making it one of Dallas's most densely packed neighborhoods, one that has encountered its share of crime and poverty over the decades.[4]

Directly down the freeway, about a five-minute drive or so, stands one of Dallas's fanciest shopping malls—in fact, it was the largest indoor shopping mall in the world when it was built in 1965. The flagship Nieman Marcus is in there (technically its second location; the first flagship closed and was moved here). It's one of those malls that has a whole wing just for couture shops that most of us mere mortals gaze at with a mix of wonder and disdain for capitalism gone so far off the deep end that $5,000 shopping bags daintily sit three minutes away from an immigrant family in a cramped apartment complex.

I personally watched as crews emptied Amber Vinson's apartment after the Presbyterian Hospital nurse also came down with Ebola. Her belongings were summarily emptied from her apartment and taken to the coast to be incinerated. At the time I was finishing my dissertation (now book) on disease and risk aversion, and I wondered what the point of all this was. As I stood among the news crews watching the "decontamination process," what I saw before me seemed to be little more than average-looking workers loading belongings into U-Haul trucks with new labels slapped on them. There didn't seem to be any special equipment involved that would limit such supposedly risky infectious particles from, say, seeping out the door or into the truck itself. No, all this really appeared to be little more than the same old story: sanitation theater, this time performed for the benefit of the wealthy citizens of

---

4   Michael E. Young, "Hope Blooms in Vickery Meadow," *Dallas Morning News Online*, January 7, 2006, https://web.archive.org/web/20071208195906/http: /www.dallasnews.com/sharedcontent/dws/news/localnews/stories/010806dnm etvickery.2a4bd98.html; and "Vickery Meadow Strategic Action Plan," Institute of Urban Studies at University of Texas, Arlington, 2017, https://issuu.com /institute-uta/docs/vickery_meadow.

Dallas, who needed to feel that something had been done about a virus when it struck close to home. Nearby, Thomas's family was ordered by a court to stay in their apartment with their dead relative's soiled linens for more than two weeks. Differences in treatment based on race, class, and gender are hardly new. Per the SSDC, these human biases are even reproduced in our fictional imaginings. And lest we forget these lessons, let us return to

LESSON 28:
What's in a name, part 2.

It's critical that *The Hot Zone* is set in an African space, not a Western one. Pushing a disease to the margins of our consciousness with fantasies of its being "natural" to a certain culture is nothing more than the same old fear-induced denial we've been talking about since **Lesson 6**. In a really provocative essay, "Dying a Natural Death: Ethics and Political Activism for Endemic Infectious Diseases," Claire Hooker, Chris Degeling, and Paul Mason make the point that even the definitions of "epidemic" (defined as an unexpected outbreak of a disease in a community) and "endemic" (defined as a disease naturally occurring at low, stable populations within a given community) are as much a representation of social factors as they are mathematical ones. For instance, Ebola is readily considered "endemic" to certain regions of West Africa. Conversely, when America encountered eleven cases within its borders, it was treated like an outbreak, whether or not it was actually called an "epidemic." The same is true of many diseases. Calling a disease "endemic" to a place makes it seem like it's okay that it's happening there, and it normalizes xenophobia by normalizing disease to "other" places and peoples. In other words, defining something as "endemic" allows us to conveniently ignore the disease and treat it as a "normal" part of a population.

If you've been following along thus far, it will come as no surprise to you that typically "endemic" diseases are identified in marginalized populations that those in power see as "Other." Ebola is "endemic" to Africa. HIV is "endemic" to the gay population. STDs are "endemic" in sex workers. Polio, we now know, was in fact universally endemic to the human population for as long as we have records of human existence—we've even found ancient Egyptian grave markers depicting people with it. But when it affected white, middle-class America, it suddenly became an "epidemic." We in the West tend to treat epidemics as unacceptable, intolerable levels of disease that must be combatted swiftly. In the case of polio, the race for the cure brought with it the game-changing polio vaccine, but how much earlier might this vaccine have been discovered had we cared about diseases of "Others" that we too readily tolerated because we treated them as natural (endemic) to that population? History bears this dynamic out time and again. Hooker, Degeling, and Mason take this so far as to say, "Viruses don't kill people—people kill people," and we do that partially through xenophobic naming practices that allow diseases to spread while we shrug our shoulders.[5]

———

Remember Kristeva from the anti-chapter? The solution to disease and death is not denial but to accept these fearful ideas and incorporate them into our minds as a part of our diverse experiences of the world. We must deeply accept, not deny, the possibility we fear. The very name *Ebola virus* marks the disease as something foreign, connected to a river in the Democratic Republic of Congo, and therefore (imaginatively and linguistically) safely away from us in the Western world.

---

5 Hooker, Degeling, and Mason, "Dying a Natural Death."

Before Ebola virus came to Dallas in 2014, West Nile virus, another disease named after a river in Africa, started making the news. Every summer night a ticker on the local news would mark the death tolls, and several times in the summer, planes sprayed pesticides over the city. I'd watch as bees and wasps lay dying on the ground, and still the WNV numbers crept up.[6] Though I least of all want to see anyone die, I found it remarkable that we Americans were willing to bomb our own environments with poison before we were willing to accept that we, too, were simply human and therefore vulnerable to infectious disease. It's remarkable, too, that while WNV is technically *endemic* to America now, it's still named after somewhere far away from us, somewhere distant and foreign.[7] *This can't have come from us*, we tell ourselves in our very naming practices. But we would do well to take heed of **Lesson 27** here. The way we talk about disease allows it to spread—especially when we're in denial.

Fortunately, it's no longer an acceptable practice to name diseases after the places of their outbreaks, because even global health organizations have finally recognized the real impact of practices like this in encouraging xenophobic attitudes. But centuries of xenophobic naming practices still linger in our medical dictionaries; the damage is done. For Priscilla Wald, the very act of trying to pinpoint a beginning point of an outbreak is itself potentially suspect.[8] In my opinion, such an epidemiological goal of finding a "source" of contagion often seems to conveniently serve those in power. If history is written by the victors, then epidemiology is written by the hegemonic majority. For all the

---

6 For a more academic take on these reflections, which I've recounted before, see my book *Kept from All Contagion*.

7 "West Nile Virus," New York State Department of Health, www.health.ny.gov /diseases/west_nile_virus/fact_sheet.htm.

8 Priscilla Wald, *Contagious: Cultures, Carriers, and the Outbreak Narrative* (Durham, NC: Duke University Press, 2008), 12.

trappings of numbers and data that seem to undergird our conclusions when the source of a disease is found, if science finds the same answer time and again, and that answer repeatedly tells us that blame never lies with us but always with foreign cultures we already distance ourselves from, we need to examine that science (**Lesson 27**). As I've said before, as a medical humanist, my job is not to rewrite these algorithms but to point out the ways in which our algorithms might be framed—intentionally or not—so as to produce a self-serving result.

Dallas, Texas
1994

I remember peering at it on my biological mother's nightstand. I hadn't ever seen her unable to stop reading before, like some insatiable, hungry animal. It was a plain white book, with an angry-looking circle emblazoned on the middle, and the simple title *The Hot Zone*. It was on the bedside table of every American housewife that summer. Perhaps it's little more than an indication I was always destined to be a literature professor specializing in infectious disease, but I have oddly vivid memories of staring at the book by her bedside, entranced. What could its contents hold that had so thoroughly hypnotized my mother?

"What's it about?" I said, sitting by her one evening while she tried to focus on reading and not on the questions I was itching to ask as they hung palpably in the air around us.

"A disease." Now I was really interested (so, yes, I guess I was always this way).

"What kind?" Here my memory lapses. I'm not sure if she told me the name of it just yet. I do remember asking for all the gory details of what the illness did to a person's body. (See? Always this way.)

"You bleed from every hole in your body."

"Every one?"

"Every single one." She turned back to her book.

"Your eyes?" I inched closer, trying to peer at the horrors, written in black and white, and translate them into my visual imagination.

"Yes." She didn't look up.

"Your nose?"

"Mm-hmm."

"Well, that's all the holes there are." Success!

She put down the book and looked at me, thinking. "Your skin has lots of tiny holes, called pores."

My eyes widened. "Do you bleed from those, too?"

"Yup. You die within twelve hours."

I don't remember the rest of the conversation precisely, but I do know that later that week, I had talked my friend next door into developing a song about what I now knew to call "Ebola" in order to educate future generations in early symptom detection. I had heard in music class that "Ring Around the Rosy" was a song describing the Black Plague, and I wanted to help out with the next big disease song. (I repeat: I was, apparently, always this way.)

I'll leave for your own discretion the consideration of whether a mother and a music teacher should have bestowed such grisly details about Ebola and the bubonic plague upon a seven-year-old, but there you have it. These moments marked me and how I thought about disease for a long, long time. What's much more important, however, is the way that *The Hot Zone* marked all of Western society.

My students leave my courses knowing it's the only book I cry over when I lecture—because, in my mind, it's fiction. At least, its depictions of Ebola and what it does to the human body are vastly inaccurate. Catherine Belling, professor of medical humanities and bioethics at Northwestern University's Feinberg School of Medicine, even notes that Charles Monet—the man whose ghastly story famously opens *The Hot Zone*—wasn't even suffering from Ebola virus; he had

Marburg hemorrhagic fever. Indeed, Belling notes that "diarrhea and vomiting, along with fever and aches, are typical, and in some cases, these excretions do contain blood. Severe hemorrhages can occur, especially in pregnant women, but the kind of explosive bleeding Preston represents is hyperbolic. He describes the appearance of symptoms in a worst-case clinical scenario."[9] These inaccuracies, combined with the book's wide circulation, created a new set of xenophobic myths about a virus, triggering the need to believe that it can't happen here, that these horrors simply won't happen to Americans. *The Hot Zone* is one of the most dangerous books ever to become a bestseller, because

LESSON 29:
Xenophobia is fear, and fear facilitates denial.

Preston's depiction of Ebola (in my view, an inaccurate and sensationalistic one) catalyzed an American fear so great that it slid easily into denial. As shown in chapter 2, risk aversion, denial, and hubris are surprisingly linked in the human psyche, one leading easily to the other in a never-ending cycle. As discussed in the anti-chapter, it is admittedly scary to truly confront the notion of our own mortality. Preston's depictions of Ebola were so extreme that Americans turned for comfort to the one constant in American disease fantasies: that fatal Western hubris that silently assures us "It won't happen here, it won't happen to us." The entire plot of *The Hot Zone*—in spite of its classification as nonfiction, it is highly editorialized—is that of a terrifying foreign disease emerging from the bowels of Africa, ultimately to be subdued by American military ingenuity. If that's not the most self-satisfied wish-fulfillment fantasy ever, I don't know what is. Remember **Lesson 14**? While disease in general causes a pen-

---

9 Belling, "Dark Zones," in *Endemic*, 37.

dulum swing of panic and denial, in a Western world where we've forgotten much of the specific horror of infectious disease, I think Preston's book is a prime example of how we've developed a zeitgeist of xenophobic panic/denialism in response to disease—one that is as self-defeating as it is bigoted. The book, I believe, aims to incite panic with images of melting flesh and contagious fluids emanating from an undifferentiated Africa (no countries necessary for this xenophobic fantasy). But remember, these are images that don't align with Ebola's actual presentation. American gumption and know-how then conquer the disease (in the book, anyway).

Should we be at all surprised, then, that when Americans heard about the novel coronavirus in China—in January 2020, before we were aware of its presence in the West—they either: (1) completely panicked before they knew much about the disease's spread, or (2) completely buried their heads in the sand? In January and February 2020, my social media feeds were filled with people masking up before the CDC formally recommended it and absolutely obsessing about not touching their faces. In other parts of my life, students were telling me about COVID-19 costume parties, where people congregated in great numbers, dressed in hospital gowns and masks, in obvious flippant disregard for a disease that was killing their fellow humans on the other side of the globe. Such behaviors are only possible when we think an issue won't affect us. Around that time, I went on the local news to share the same lesson I'm sharing with you here: We can't live in fear *or* denial. The only certainty we have is that disease *will* spread to all the hosts it can, and if we can embrace this reality, we can work together with all our global citizen-neighbors to combat it. If we do otherwise, we're simply its next victims.

The legacy of Ebola in America began in 1994 when Preston's book was published. But it continued on in the legacy of the novel coronavirus (foregrounded by the histories of syphilis and HIV), and it makes it clear that the more we think "not us," the more we give pathogens a chance to spread and wind up right at our doorstep.

The seemingly mischaracterized aspects of Ebola in *The Hot Zone*, to my thinking, still cause revulsion and panic in response to the word today, particularly when we hear it in the news. As I'll explain momentarily, I firmly believe that this fear reaction, cultivated (in my opinion) by Preston's book, is a huge problem, not only for our collective cultural attitudes but also for our bodies. In other words, I think *The Hot Zone*, a little paperback written almost twenty-eight years ago, has real effects on our abilities to contain pandemics today, not only because of the dynamics outlined in **Lesson 27** but also because

LESSON 30:
Prejudice is a disease.

Or perhaps, to put it more accurately, prejudice allows disease to spread. Again, this chapter may feel a bit repetitive, but I find that these lessons are worth repeating because they are the hardest zeitgeists to recognize and therefore to shirk. When we believe we are somehow immune from a disease because of a social characteristic of ours—our nationality, for instance—we engage in a belief that means absolutely nothing to a microbiological pathogen. It simply makes us sitting ducks, moved to denial through our fear, and consequently not taking definitive action against the pathogen in community with others. As I've said repeatedly in this book, disease unites us all, whether we like to think so or not, and when we refuse to believe this, disease only unites us further in shared death. Our very fear of death (recall the anti-chapter) motivates us to believe that any small difference (sexuality, lifestyle, class) might save us, but this fantasy in fact only opens the floodgates for more pathogenic spread as we saunter around in self-satisfied delusion. As far as viruses and bacteria go, we have two options, and two options alone: we can live together—and I mean really live together, working toward equality between the underdeveloped and developed worlds and caring for our neighbors' health as we would our own—or we can die together. It's all the same to a virus. If it makes any difference to us, we must act.

CONCLUSION

COVID-19'S DARKEST TIMELINE

(and How to Reverse Course)

———

How do you end a book on plague when you're in the middle of the plague, and I, no more than anyone, have any clue how it will end? We accept the many, many uncertainties and sort through the wreckage of the lives that we knew to find the few certainties we think we can still count on.

Here's what I know: at the time of writing this, in a landscape that is changing by the day, this will be dated by the time you read it, but the conclusions, no matter when you read them, hold true. This could still go so many ways. We aren't out of the woods yet, in terms of how many human lives will be touched by this viral pathogen. By the time my revisions to this book were due just eight weeks after finishing the main draft, the landscape had vastly changed, and the pandemic had become worse than ever. Even once it's winding down, we won't be out of the woods. It will be years before we know how the human reactions to this virus will impact our psyches for the rest of our lives, as well as the toll it may take on future generations. Children and grandchildren of people who lived through America's Great Depression felt the effects for decades and decades after the Depression itself ended—the emphasis on saving everything, parental decrees to clean all the food on plates, an intrinsic belief that more must be better, because having nothing had been so very traumatic—these are behaviors we're still sorting through in 2020. Shows like *Hoarders*, American obesity numbers (and the concomitant fat-shaming movement, which is perhaps more horrific), and conspicuous consumption of material goods that none of us need are all partially aftereffects of a generation long before us that was impacted by the sudden, extreme poverty experienced almost a century ago. What will a year of school closings do not just to *our* children but to *their* children? And *their* children? What has the ever-increasing divide between our ability to find commonalities with our fellow man done to our hearts? To politics? To religious movements? Even once the biological hazard of the virus passes, humanity will see ripple effects of the COVID-19 pandemic long after anyone reading this book is dead. In fact, as I'm reviewing the final manuscript in February 2021, we don't seem to be able to see the end of the pandemic yet; perhaps the disease will be known as the 2020 pandemic in the same way that the 1918 flu pandemic clung to its nominal year, even as it spanned several. My point is this: when I started writing this book in 2020, the idea that this pandemic would remain relegated to 2020 seemed reasonable. Today, in 2021, I've given up on even estimating when this will all end. So even if you're reading this in 2022 or 2030, there's still work to do.

———

I also know that when things are indeterminate, when a situation could still go many ways, that sometimes horrifying uncertainty also means we still have a fighting chance, even if we feel too tired to keep fighting.

But please keep fighting.

Viruses don't tire. They've got an edge on us in that way. But they don't have human ingenuity and grit. They can't *care* about what they've got to lose the way we do. That's our edge—we have the motivation and drive to look at the world around us and decide to save it.

I know you're tired. I'm tired. But I wrote this book for you—to help give you hope by providing you with a list of strategies so that you can keep fighting when you want to lay down your defenses, and when giving up seems like a balmy sort of rest compared to sticking it out and working toward a hopeful horizon that seems to recede by the second.

———

Here's what else I know. I know what we need to do to win. I know how we find ourselves again even once this particular virus no longer threatens us, as we struggle to secure a foothold in "normal," and as we prepare for the inevitable next virus that we, or our children, or our children's children face (for you are the child's child's child of someone who survived the 1918 pandemic, and whoever they were, they wanted you—the mere wisp of a fancy of an idea of their continued legacy on this planet—to make it). So, here's how we make it: **community, creativity, and communication.**

Every lesson in this book has been one key part of developing these three values and practices. They've been quick and specific tips for working these things into your daily life. They've been a how-to guide for coping with and thinking through specific problems that have come up for many people in 2020, based on what I have learned are predictable issues in times of disease outbreak. But I can't possibly cover every contingency or situation, of course. For that reason, it's important to leave you with the general formula for success so that you can apply it to everything you do, everywhere you look, and everyone you talk with, even issues that may be unforeseen as of yet, or things I simply couldn't cover directly here.

COMMUNITY.

I've said this a few times now, but the best part of disease is that it forces us to realize we *are* in community with one another, whether we like it or not. It calls our bluff on all the false differences we've erected between ourselves—like class, race, sexuality, and nationality—that we think separate us, and that, in many cases, people use to justify their superiority over others. We're all in this together, even if some of us choose to believe otherwise. Whether we choose to play on the same team or not, we're all necessarily in the same game. Biologically, we are yoked by our humanness to one another, and we all exist together amid a sea of invisible particles that make their way in life by feeding on us. *All* of us. Left unchecked, the very privileges that allow those in power to imagine themselves outside of this community—as somehow immune to disease, that is—will in fact be the things that allow a disease to spread so much that it eventually destroys us all. Because viruses don't care about our money and our privilege, they just need time to spread while we fool ourselves into believing we're not all part of the same human buffet the virus needs to survive.

To be clear, there will always be those who cannot accept our common community as humans. But the more of us who can accept it—and I mean radically accept it, by communing with our opponents and working toward connecting—the stronger we all are against viral and bacterial pathogens. When we divide ourselves, we've already done half the work of "dividing and conquering" for the microbes—that buffet becomes a free lunch, and pathogens can simply swoop in for the kill. The more of us who fight the good fight of acknowledging and celebrating our community, of building bridges between perceived division, of fighting racism, transphobia, sex-worker phobia, and wage slavery, the harder we make it for disease to conquer us. Remember: they are mere algorithms. *We* contain multitudes.

CREATIVITY.

It's going to take radical forms of community for us to learn all we can, to brainstorm every means of fighting the virus, and, equally as important, to cope with its psychosocial impacts as we take precautions to stay safe. It's not always an either/or of lockdown or total disregard for safety. Together, we can find balance in a middle ground that protects us while allowing us to live full lives within the community that we so desperately need. And the answers about where this path lies and how to find it are not going to come just from the scientists and professors. How about the cholera outbreak John Snow investigated? Better sewage drainage built into city infrastructure was a key part of the solution. What about later typhoid outbreaks near the end of the century? Plumbing innovation solved that problem.

Seriously; my friend Christian Alvarez, who is a plumber, recently said to me in passing, "The p-trap was the greatest invention ever for modern plumbing."[1] And he's right. The concept foregrounding the use of the p-trap (a design in piping that allows for ventilation in such a way that sewer gases don't back up) was a Victorian-era idea. The Victorians realized that ventilated pipes counterintuitively allowed for a more efficient means of moving sewage material and gases away from family homes and into sewers where they could be contained and broken down by probiotic processes—which, by the way, Victorians also capitalized on, and which we still use as an integral part of septic systems. A plumber or an HVAC technician could very well be an important part of solving the issues we're facing today as well. We won't know unless we put our heads together and talk and think in community.

---

1 Christian Alvarez, personal communication.

In 2012, my friend Preston Benson, who is now a pastor but was once a prison administrator, was part of a Forward Thinking Team organized to develop innovative, proactive solutions for prisons and our society. While on that team, he suggested that labor in prisons should be put toward making PPE and medical packaging for single-dose pharmaceuticals.[2] His thinking was that this might prevent American overreliance on such vital products from overseas, in case such supply chains became disrupted—say, in the event of a pandemic. His idea wasn't taken up at the time because of political infighting in DC, but what if it had been? A prison administrator had an idea years before that could have been a 2020 game-changer before we even knew we needed a game-changer. My point is that scientists are part of the solution, but the solutions are going to cross many disciplines and walks of life. If plumbers and correctional officers have had ideas with the potential to actually save us from infectious disease, imagine all the different people who might have ideas to get schools safely going again. Or to actually implement contactless delivery at an affordable rate for everyone so that workers and consumers are protected. Or to stimulate the postal service, which has become more important than ever during quarantine. The answers are going to come from everywhere, and they are going to draw from the rich experiences that you don't even yet realize the people all around you have. Which brings me to

COMMUNICATION.

Just think about it. The person bagging your groceries probably notices small inefficiencies in their daily job that corporate employees never get on the ground floor to see. Have you ever actually spoken with people in hotel housekeeping about which surfaces they think

---

2   Reverend Preston Benson, personal communication.

are the hardest to clean? Have you asked public-school teachers about the subtle ways Zoom chat rooms are allowing quiet kids to chime in more readily? We've got to talk to each other, hungrily and constantly. We have to try to learn from experiences we might never have—that we might not even realize we don't have—and utilize the expertise that *each and every one of us* has, even if in a small realm of our lives. Only through communication can we draw from the **creative** ideas we would never otherwise know our neighbor had, and then, in the **community** we've created with **communication**, work together to implement and build such solutions. The critical thinking tips in this book are what I have to offer, but the pragmatic answers hardly lie with me. My creative gift is pinpointing communication gaps, and I hope that by offering these insights to you, you will find the strength to carry on when you're tired and to build the community that somewhere— probably somewhere we haven't even thought of—has the solutions to build a better world for us.

Victorian poet Alfred, Lord Tennyson, wrote a poem in 1832 (around the time of the Sunderland cholera epidemic featured in chapter 3) called "The Lady of Shalott." In the poem, Tennyson invents a myth that he sets in medieval times and is entirely fictional. In this poem, an otherwise unnamed lady (the Lady of Shalott) is stuck in a tower, cursed.

Bear with me here, because her curse is a little . . . weird. She is cursed not only to stay in the tower but also, if she so much as looks out the window (and there is, of course, a window to tempt her), she'll die. So, as a sort of loophole, she spends her days with a mirror set up angled toward the window, allowing her to see reflections of what's out there in the world. And she weaves a tapestry of all she sees.

But the poem isn't actually about her looking into a mirror and weaving. No sooner than we're given this setup, the Lady of Shalott declares, "I am Half-sick of Shadows," and looks out the window.

No hero comes to save her. No secret trick breaks the curse.

Nope, she definitely dies.

But . . . why? Why am I sitting here, at the end of a book about how history can help us learn how to survive disease, telling you about some made-up lady who died a made-up death in a poem that's over a century old?

Well, I love this poem, because the main character chooses real-world experiences—to really live—rather than staying in her room and continuing to merely exist. The reason she looks out the window and then leaves her tower is important; she sees another human, and she craves human connection.

She would rather die than not experience that. For her, the world of "shadows" doesn't count as a meaningful life, and it's worth it to her to trade in one moment of really living for a lifetime of safety. Safety is, well, safe, but really it's a guaranteed life of stagnation and isolation.

Of course, I'm asking you to consider this metaphorically, because although I've said much about risk mitigation (versus elimination) and acceptance of our mortality in this book, none of us wants to die, nor should we. Let me be clear once more: I'm an advocate of moderation, and that means both taking precautions *and* accepting that risk is inevitable. I do not mean we should literally throw caution to the wind and ignore public health recommendations entirely to follow the Lady of Shalott's example. Because, of course, Tennyson's poem is a fictional scenario, and fiction allows authors to use ideas like death to make important points not just about literal death but also about how they think we should live our inevitably finite *lives*.

In my opinion, Tennyson very much meant for us to read the poem metaphorically, because the poem itself is really quite silly when taken literally, even given its imaginary medieval setting. For one, most of his "medieval"-style poems are based in actual medieval legends, whereas this one is entirely made up. It feels a little out of place, like a break in the pattern of his typical work. And because he's simply made it up, there's no way to justify the very odd "curse" as part of legend or tradition.

Why can't she look out the window anyway? And how exactly does looking out the window through a mirror not "count" as breaking the curse?

Again, if this were ancient folklore, we'd probably give it a pass. Arthur's grail is holy . . . well, because it is. Cupid's arrow makes two people fall in love . . . because it does. But Katniss Everdeen better have a backstory to make us believe that she can shoot an arrow.

The fact that this poem doesn't make a lot of intuitive sense, the fact that we just have to accept the rules of the game as Tennyson sets them up and sit with our uncomfortable questions about his dubious world-building, all from a poet who usually played by the rules of composition—for me, it means this is all meant to be taken as high metaphor.

Remember: the Lady of Shalott is an artist—she weaves tapestries of the world she sees.

So why does she quit?

I would argue that this is because, as I've hinted, she wants more. She knows that her life is no life at all, and—here is where I see the connection to our lives even today—she knows that she can't "write" in her tapestry of life without having really lived it.

She declares boldly that she is "half-sick of shadows"—that is, she no longer thinks it's enough to passively observe life at a distance and simply "reflect" what she sees—doubly through the mirror and in her copies of it in thread.

Instead, she decides that ultimately, to represent life in her art, she must go live it boldly, whatever the cost (and her cost is indeed high, making Tennyson's point quite clear).

I say this a lot in my classes, and it feels like something of a bold statement, but I've yet to find an example of it not being true: our deepest moments of learning do not occur where we're comfortable.

We're comfortable with what we know. We're comfortable with what we're used to. That comfort, by definition, does not add to or challenge the world as we know it. Deep, meaningful moments of learning and growth cause discomfort. They often happen in our lowest lows. But sometimes this just means that we're challenged to question a belief we've always had or an assumption we didn't realize we built long ago.

The Lady of Shalott is comfortable in her tower. But there's no growth there. And, importantly, she realizes that this lack of growth is an intellectual and emotional death. She *must* face danger, risk, and discomfort if she is to grow and truly live. So, here's my parting charge to those of you looking for concrete ways to help fix things:

Go outside your comfort zone. Have a cup of coffee with *that person* (you know who I'm talking about) whose political ideas make you see red. And just . . . *talk*. Remind yourself that they are a human with needs, values, and fears like your own. That they, too, love their children and fear for them. That their anger, like yours, comes from a place of insecurity, doubt, and desire for a better world. Because the more I've talked with people while writing this book—hairdressers, colleagues, friends, strangers—the more I'm convinced that the differences I see on the surface are red herrings meant to divide us, to distract us from the ways we could be banding together. Believe me, I'm strongly, perhaps aggressively political, and I get angry, too. But I've found that when I can lay aside those feelings and talk to those who are supposed to be my enemies—really talk with them and allow them space for feelings that make me uncomfortable and views that seem patently and obviously inaccurate—I find that they are human like me, just a speck in a vast universe trying to make sense of chaos . . . like me. Now, I do draw the line at humanitarian issues, and I won't tolerate others speaking of other humans as if they don't have rights and intrinsic value. *But* (and it feels weird to say "but" here) how can I convince people effectively to change their human rights attitudes if I can't have a conversation with them to begin with? So, start small. Have the cup of coffee. Shake the hand (or fist-bump, whatever social-distancing practices require). Acknowledge disagreement, but actively meet it with openness and curiosity, even when you want to dig your heels in and fire back retorts. Have the conversation that you're scared to have.

Because outside of our normal is challenging, invigorating life.

And in open, engaged, earnest communication—communication that seeks to understand, not always yet to persuade—we find the seeds of community and creativity that just might save us all.

BIBLIOGRAPHY

- ABC News. "Ebola-Stricken Surgeon Martin Salia Died Despite ZMapp, Plasma Transfusion." ABC News, November 17, 2104. https://abcnews.go.com/Health/ebola-stricken-surgeon-martin-salia-died-zmapp-plasma/story?id=26964778.

- "A Brief History of Handwashing." *The Week*, no. 1272 (2020), 55.

- Acton, William. *The Contagious Disease Acts: Shall the Contagious Disease Acts Be Applied to the Civil Population?* London: John Churchill and Sons, 1870.

- Adams, Clifford, Anne Lavin, Anne van Dyke, Elizabeth Struchesky, and Louise Abruchezze. "'Please, Let Me Put Him in a Macaroni Box': The Spanish Influenza of 1918 in Philadelphia." Interview by Charles Hardy, WHYY-FM radio. History Matters: The U.S. Survey Course on the Web. http://historymatters.gmu.edu/d/13.

- "The Address by Which M. Pasteur." *London Evening Standard*, May 1, 1882, p. 7.

- Agamben, Giorgio. *Homo Sacer: Sovereign Power and Bare Life.* Stanford. CA: Stanford University Press, 1995.

- Ahern, Laurie. "Orphanages Are No Place for Children." *Washington Post*, August 9, 2013. www.washingtonpost.com/opinions/orphanages-are-no-place-for-children/2013/08/09/6d502fb0-fadd-11e2-a369-d1954abcb7e3_story.html.

- Ai, Jong-Wen, QiauLing Ruan, Qi-Hui Liu, and Wen-Hong Zhang. "Updates on the Risk Factors for Latent Tuberculosis Reactivation and their Managements." *Emerging Microbes and Infections* 5, no. 2 (2016): 10.

- Ainsworth, W. "Observations on the Pestilential Cholera (Asphyxia Pestilenta), as It Appeared at Sunderland in the Months of November and December 1831; and on the Measures Taken for Its Prevention and Cure." *London Literary Gazette* 18 (1832): 97.

- Ainsworth, W. "Original Correspondence: Cholera." *Literary Gazette* (1832): 601.

- "Alice L. Mikel Duffield." *Veterans History Project*. Library of Congress, October 26, 2011. https://memory.loc.gov/diglib/vhp/story/loc.natlib.afc2001001.01747/?loclr=blogflt.

- Allen, Michelle. "From Cesspool to Sewer: Sanitary Reform and the Rhetoric of Resistance, 1848–1880." *Victorian Literature and Culture* 30, no. 2 (2002): 393.

- Alvarez, Christian. Personal communication.

- *American Influenza Epidemic of 1918–1919: A Digital Encyclopedia.* www.influenzaarchive.org.

- American Society for Microbiology. "C. Difficile Resists Hospital Disinfectant, Persists on Hospital Gowns, Stainless Steel." *EurekAlert!*,

July 12, 2019. www.eurekalert.org/pub_releases/2019-07/asfm-cdr 070919.php.

- "Another Book on Bacteriology." *Saturday Review*, August 1, 1891.

- "Appeal to Ignorance." Texas State University: Department of Philosophy. www.txstate.edu/philosophy/resources/fallacy-definitions /Appeal-to-Ignorance.html.

- Archer, Johnny. "Eric Duncan's Fiancee Struggles to Rebuild Life." *NBCDFW*, October 30, 2014. www.nbcdfw.com/news/local/eric -duncans-fiance-talks-to-nbc-5/1992118/.

- Arnold, Carrie. "The Viruses That Made Us Human." *NOVA*, September 28, 2016.

- Associated Press. "After the Quarantine: 'I Want to Breathe.'" *Politico*, October 19, 2014. www.politico.com/story/2014/10 /ebola-thomas-duncan-girlfriend-louise-troh-112013.

- Bailey-Denton, E. *Sewage Purification Brought Up to Date*. New York: Spon and Chamberlain, 1896.

- Barnes, David. *The Great Stink of Paris and the Nineteenth-Century Struggle against Filth and Germs*. Baltimore: Johns Hopkins University Press, 2006.

- Barnes, Diana. "The Public Life of a Woman of Wit and Quality: Lady Mary Wortley Montagu and the Vogue for Smallpox Inoculation." *Feminist Studies* 38 (2012): 330–62.

- "The Battle of the Bacilli." *The Outlook*, December 30, 1899.

- Bazin, Herve. *Vaccination: A History from Lady Montagu to Genetic Engineering*. Montrouge: John Libby, 2011.

- Beaubien, Jason. "Fond Memories of Ebola Victim Eric Duncan, Anger over His Death." *Morning Edition*, NPR, October 9, 2014.

- Bell, Ian A. *Defoe's Fiction*. London: Croom Helm, 1985.

- Belling, Catherine. "Dark Zones: The Ebola Body as a Configuration of Horror." *Essays in Contagion Theory*. London: Palgrave, 2016: 43–66.

- Benson, Reverend Preston. Personal communication.

- Benton, Adia. *HIV Exceptionalism: Development through Disease in Sierra Leone*. Minneapolis: University of Minnesota Press, 2015.

- Berlinger, Nancy, et al. "Ethical Framework for Health Care Institutions & Guidelines for Institutional Ethics Services Responding to the Coronavirus Pandemic: Managing Uncertainty, Safeguarding Communities, Guiding Practice." Hastings Center, March 16, 2020. www.thehastingscenter.org/ethicalframeworkcovid19/.

- Best, M., D. Neuhauser, and L. Slavin. "'Cotton Mather, You Dog, Dam You! I'l Inoculate You with this; With a Pox to You': Smallpox Inoculation, Boston, 1721." *Quality and Safety in Health Care* 13 (2004): 82–83.

- Bewell, Alan. *Romanticism and Colonial Disease*. Baltimore: Johns Hopkins University Press, 1999.

- Bilson, Andy. "The Babies Who Suffer in Silence: How Overseas Orphanages Are Damaging Children." *The Telegraph*, November 6,

2017. www.telegraph.co.uk/health-fitness/body/babies-suffer-silence
-overseas-orphanages-damaging-children/.

- Bissell, Helen W. "Health, Beauty, and the Toilet." *Bow Bells*, August 19, 1892.

- Bochner, Salomon. *The Role of Mathematics in the Rise of Science*. Princeton, NJ: Princeton University Press, 1966.

- Bodkin, Christopher. "Superbugs Cling to Hospital Gowns Even after They Have Been Disinfected." *The Telegraph*, July 12, 2019. www.telegraph.co.uk/science/2019/07/12/superbugs-cling -hospital-gowns-even-have-disinfected/.

- Boiocchi, Federica, Matthew P. Davies, and Anthony C. Hilton. "An Examination of Flying Insects in Seven Hospitals in the United Kingdom and Carriage of Bacteria by True Flies (Diptera: Calliphoridae, Dolichopodidae, Fanniidae, Muscidae, Phoridae, Psychodidae, Sphaeroceridae)," *Journal of Medical Entomology* 56, no. 6 (2019): 1684–97. https://doi.org/10.1093/jme/tjz086.

- Botelho, Greg, and Jacque Wilson. "Thomas Eric Duncan: First Ebola Death in U.S.," CNN, October 8, 2014. www.cnn.com /2014/10/08/health/thomas-eric-duncan-ebola/index.html.

- Brantley, Ann, ed. "1918 Pandemic Influenza Survivors Share Their Stories." Alabama Public Health, April 14, 2017. https://www .alabamapublichealth.gov/pandemicflu/1918-influenza-survivor -stories.html.

- "The Bristol Mob." *The Examiner* 19 (1832): 540.

- "The Broad Street Pump." *The Examiner* (1855): 738.

- Brodsky, Phyllis L. *The Control of Childbirth: Women versus Medicine through the Ages*. Jefferson: McFarland, 2008.

- Brodsley, Laurel. "Defoe's *The Journal of the Plague Year*: A Model for Stories of Plagues." In *AIDS: The Literary Response*, edited by Emmanuel S. Nelson, 11–22. New York: Twayne, 1992.

- Brody, Howard, Michael Russell Rip, Peter Vinten-Johansen, Nigel Paneth, and Stephen Rachman. "Map-making and Myth-making in Broad Street: The London Cholera Epidemic, 1854." *The Lancet* 351, no. 9223 (2000): 64–68.

- Bruininks, Patricia. E-mail correspondence, August 18, 2020; August 21, 2020; and September 17, 2020.

- Bulteel, Christopher. *Contagious Disease Acts Considered in their Moral, Social, and Sanitary Aspects*. London: Robert Hardwicke, 1870.

- Burnett, Paul. "Dying by Inches: Epidemics and Oral History." Berkeley Library, April 9, 2020. https://update.lib.berkeley.edu /2020/04/09/dying-by-inches-epidemics-and-oral-history/.

- Bynum, Helen. *Spitting Blood: The History of Tuberculosis*. Oxford, UK: Oxford University Press, 2012.

- Bynum, W. F. "In Retrospect: On the Mode of Communication of Cholera." *Nature* 495, no. 7440 (2013): 169–70.

- ———. *Science and the Practice of Medicine in the Nineteenth Century*. Cambridge, UK: Cambridge University Press, 1994.

- Byrne, Katherine. *Tuberculosis and the Victorian Literary Imagination.* Cambridge, UK: Cambridge University Press, 2013.

- Campbell, William. "Letter to Dr. R. Lee." *London Medical Gazette,* December 10, 1831, 353.

- ———. *A Treatise on the Epidemic Puerperal Fever.* Edinburgh: Bell and Bradfute, 1822.

- Cañete, Pablo F., and Carola G. Vinuesa. "COVID-19 Makes B Cells Forget, but T Cells Remember." *Cell* 183 (2020): 13–15.

- "Carbolic Smoke Ball." *Strand Magazine,* January 1892, 20.

- "Carbolic Smoke Ball." *Tinsleys' Magazine,* July 1889.

- Cardoso Leão, Sylvia, Maria Isabel Romano, and Maria Jesus Garcia. "Tuberculosis, Leprosy, and Other Mycobacterioses." *Bioinformatics in Tropical Disease Research: A Practical and Case-Study Approach* (2006).

- Carpenter, W. B. "The Germ-Theory of Zymotic Diseases: Considered from the Natural History Point of View." *The Nineteenth-Century: A Monthly Review,* February 1884.

- Centers for Disease Control and Prevention. "Pandemic Influenza Storybook." www.cdc.gov/publications/panflu/index.html.

- ———. "TB Risk Factors." www.cdc.gov/tb/topic/basics/risk.htm.

- ———. "What Is Ebola Virus Disease?" Ebola (Ebola Virus Disease), n.d. www.cdc.gov/vhf/ebola/about.html.

- Chai, Qiyao, Yong Zhang, and Cui Hua Liu. "*Mycobacterium tuberculosis*: An Adaptable Pathogen Associated with Multiple Human Diseases." *Frontiers in Cellular and Infection Microbiology* 8 (2018): 158.

- Chang, Kimberly S. G. "The Hidden Pandemic Behind COVID-19." Health Resources and Services Administration, June 2020. www.hrsa.gov/enews/past-issues/2020/june-18/hidden-pandemic.

- Chapple, J. A. V. *Science and Literature in the Nineteenth Century.* Hampshire, UK: Macmillan, 1986.

- Chatburn, Andi, DO, MA, HEC-C. Personal communication.

- Chavez, Stella M. "In Vickery Meadow, Ebola's Epicenter, Life Returns to Normal." KERA Breakthroughs, 2017. http://stories.kera .org/surviving-ebola/2015/09/05/vickery-meadow-one-year-later/.

- Cheriyedath, Susha. "Most COVID-19 Convalescent Individuals Have Long-Lasting Memory T-Cell Responses." News Medical Life Sciences, November 18, 2020. www.news-medical.net/news /20201118/Most-COVID-19-convalescent-individuals-have-long -lasting-memory-T-cell-responses.aspx.

- Choi, Charles Q. "Mysterious 'Fats Radio Bursts' Fire Rhythmically through the Cosmos, Study Finds." Space.com, June 17, 2020. www.space.com/fast-radio-bursts-rhythm-discovery.html.

- "Cholera and Cholera Scares." *Saturday Review* (1884): 19.

- Christensen, Allan Conrad. *Nineteenth-Century Narratives of Contagion: "Our Feverish Contact."* London: Routledge, 2005.

- "Clarke's Blood Mixture." *Gentleman's Magazine*, December 1896.

- Clements, Jessica, and Kari Nixon. *Optimal Motherhood and Other Lies Facebook Told Us: Assembling the Networked Ethos of Contemporary Maternity Advice*. Cambridge, MA: MIT University Press, forthcoming.

- Cole, Lucinda. "The Raw, the Cooked, and the Scavenged: Beasts of the Southern Wild." *Journal for Critical Animal Studies* 12 (2014): 136–47.

- "Consumption." *Chambers's Edinburgh Journal*, October 3, 1835.

- *The Contagious Diseases Acts: Or, a Few Suggestions for Controlling Men as Well As Women*. London: 1873.

- Cooke, Jennifer. "Writing Plague: Transforming Narrative, Witnessing, and History." In *The Tapestry of Health, Illness, and Disease*, edited by Peter L. Twohig and Vera Kalizkus, 21–42. Amsterdam: Rodopi, 2008.

- "Coronavirus Death Toll." Worldometer, n.d. www.worldometers .info/coronavirus/coronavirus-death-toll/.

- Cuffari, Benedette. "The Size of SARS-CoV-2 Compared to Other Things." News Medical Life Sciences, July 16, 2020. www.news -medical.net/health/The-Size-of-SARS-CoV-2-Compared-to -Other-Things.aspx.

- "The Cure of Consumption: By One Who Has Been Cured." *Pall Mall*, June 1903.

- Czuczka, Tony, and Yuegi Yang. "Virus Fatigue Is Risk as U.S. Heads into Fall, Ex-FDA Head Says." *Bloomberg*, September 6, 2020. www.bloomberg.com/news/articles/2020-09-06/virus-fatigue-is -risk-as-u-s-heads-into-fall-ex-fda-head-says.

- D'Accolti, Maria, Irene Soffritti, Sante Mazzacane, and Elizabeth Caselli. "Fighting AMR in the Healthcare Environment: Microbiome-Based Sanitation Approaches and Monitoring Tools." *International Journal of Molecular Sciences* 20, no. 7 (2019): 1535.

- Dahlstrom, M. F. "Using Narratives and Storytelling to Communicate Science with Nonexpert Audiences." *Proceedings of the National Academy of Sciences of the United States of America* 111, no. S4 (2014): 13614–20. https://doi.org/10.1073/pnas.1320645111.

- Dale, William. *A Popular, Non-Technical, Treatise on Consumption, with Remarks on Infection, Heredity, Causes, etc.* Harrogate: R. Ackrill, 1884.

- Dalrymple, Theodore. "Unsyphilised Behaviour." *British Medical Journal*, August 21, 2010.

- Davies, David. "Successful Disinfection." In *Medical and Other Uses of Carbolic Acid.* Manchester: F. C. Calvert. Reprint of letter dated 1867.

- Day, Carolyn. *The Consumptive Chic: A History of Beauty, Fashion, and Disease.* New York: Bloomsbury, 2017.

- Defoe, Daniel. *The Complete English Tradesman.* London: Charles Rivington, 1727.

- ———. *Due Preparations for the Plague, as Well for Soul as Body.* London: J.M. Dent & Co., 1895.

- ———. *A Journal of the Plague Year.* Oxford: Oxford University Press, 1998.

- ———. *Review.* New York: Columbia University Press, 1938.

- DeGabriele, Peter. "Intimacy, Survival, and Resistance: Daniel Defoe's 'A Journal of the Plague Year,'" *ELH* 77, no. 1 (2010): 1–23.

- Delasco. "Safety Data Sheet." www.delasco.com/content/sds/PHEN OL_1-SDS.pdf.

- Derrida, Jacques. *Of Grammatology.* Baltimore: Johns Hopkins University Press, 1974.

- "Descovy for PrEP Commercial." Zheng Wen, January 30, 2020. YouTube video, 1:29. www.youtube.com/watch?v=nhsF7Csninw.

- Devereaux, Bret. Twitter thread, August 18, 2020, https://twitter .com/BretDevereaux/.

- Diamond, Dan. "Ebola's Incredibly Infectious. Ebola's Also Hard to Catch. Confused? Here's How to Understand." *Forbes*, October 16, 2014. www.forbes.com/sites/dandiamond/2014/10/16/ebolas -very-contagious-ebolas-also-hard-to-catch-confused-heres-how -to-understand/?sh=12a7ff5a5b60.

- DiBacco, Thomas V. "Childbed Fever and Hand Washing." *Washington Post*, March 23, 1993. www.washingtonpost.com/archive/lifestyle

/wellness/1993/03/23/childbed-fever-and-hand-washing/a1b3b0ee
-4b46-41ee-be37-170de0bb615b.

- Dijkstra, Bram. *Defoe and Economics: The Fortunes of Roxana in the History of Interpretation.* New York: St. Martin's Press, 1987.

- The Truth About TB. "Do I Have TB?" TB Alert, n.d. www.thetruth abouttb.org/do-i-have-tb/.

- Dong, Tao. "Persistent Immune Memory of COVID-19 Found in Recovered Patient T-Cells." *University of Oxford News,* September 4, 2020. www.ox.ac.uk/news/2020-09-04-persistent-immune-memory -covid-19-found-recovered-patient-t-cells-0.

- Dorn, Andrew. "Here's Why People Care Less as More People Die and How that Impacts the COVID-19 Pandemic." KGW8, August 11, 2020. www.kgw.com/article/tech/science/psychic-numbing-why -we-stop-caring/283-35da22bd-0fc3-4880-909b-8b3c4053476a.

- Douglas, Mary. *Purity and Danger.* New York: Routledge, 1966.

- Douglass, William. *A Dissertation Concerning Inoculation of the Small-Pox.* Boston: Henchman, 1730.

- "Doulton's Germ-Proof Filter." Advertisement, *The Sphere* 33 (1908): xi.

- Dowling, Linda. *Hellenism and Homosexuality in Victorian Oxford.* Ithaca, NY: Cornell University Press, 1997.

- Downes, Arthur Henry. *How to Avoid Typhoid Fever.* London: 1876.

- Dubos, Rene, and Jean Dubos. *The White Plague: Tuberculosis, Man, and Society.* New Brunswick, NJ: Rutgers University Press, 1987.

- Duffield, Alice L. "Interview with Alice L. Duffield." Interview by Linda Barnickel, Veterans History Project, Library of Congress, March 4, 2002, https://memory.loc.gov/diglib/vhp/story/loc.natlib.afc2001001.01747/transcript?ID=sr0001.

- Duncan, James. "Illustrations of Infantile Pathology: No. II. Measles." From *The Dublin Journal of Medical Science*, 1842, housed at the Wellcome Library Digital Collections, https://wellcomelibrary.org/item/b21913110#?c=0&m=0&s=0&cv=2&z=0.0274%2C0.5779%2C0.8524%2C0.4313&r=0.

- Durbach, Nadja. *Bodily Matters: The Anti-Vaccination Movement in England, 1853–1907*. Durham, NC: Duke University Press, 2004.

- Dye, Nancy Schrom. "The Medicalization of Birth." In *The American Way of Birth*, edited by Pamela S. Eakins, 21–46. Philadelphia: Temple University Press, 1986.

- Dyer, Carol A. *Tuberculosis*. Santa Barbara: Greenwood, 2010.

- Eakins, Pamela S., ed. *The American Way of Birth*. Philadelphia: Temple University Press, 1986.

- "Early Childhood Development and COVID-19." UNICEF, April 2020, https://data.unicef.org/topic/early-childhood-development/covid-19/.

- "Early Life on Earth—Animal Origins." National Museum of Natural History, https://naturalhistory.si.edu/education/teaching-resources/life-science/early-life-earth-animal-origins.

- "The Ebola Alarmists." *The Economist*, October 13, 2014. www.economist.com/united-states/2014/10/13/the-ebola-alarmists.

- Elbagir, Nima, and Ben Brumfield. "Back in Liberia, Ebola Is Killing Thomas Duncan's Neighbors." CNN, October 6, 2014.

- Ellison, Katherine E. *Fatal News: Reading and Information Overload in Early Eighteenth-Century Literature.* New York: Routledge, 2006.

- "Enamel Soil Pipe." Advertisement, in *Lectures on Sanitary Plumbing.* London: Haldane, 1891–92.

- Eno's Fruit Salt. *Longman's Magazine,* November 1897.

- Epstein, Steven. *Impure Science: AIDS, Activism and the Politics of Knowledge.* Berkeley: University of California Press, 1996.

- Esfandiary, Helen. "'We Could Not Answer to Ourselves Not Doing It': Maternal Obligations and Knowledge of Smallpox Inoculation in Eighteenth-Century Elite Society." *Historical Research* 92 (2019): 754–70.

- "Everything You Need to Know About OCD in the Age of COVID-19." McLean Hospital, October 4, 2020. www.mcleanhospital.org/essential/living-ocd-during-coronavirus-crisis.

- "Family Exposed to Ebola Patient Is Moved While Cleanup Continues." *Dallas Morning News,* October 4, 2014. www.dallasnews.com/news/2014/10/04/family-exposed-to-ebola-patient-is-moved-while-cleanup-continues/.

- Farr, William. *Report on the Mortality of Cholera in England, 1848–49.* London: Clowes and Sons, 1852, plate 4.

- Feldberg, Georgina. *Disease and Class: Tuberculosis and the Shaping of Modern North American Society.* New Brunswick, NJ: Rutgers University Press, 1995.

- Finger, Anne. *Elegy for a Disease: A Personal and Cultural History of Polio.* New York: St. Martin's Press, 2013.

- Fischer, Molly. "Maybe It's Lyme: What Happens When Illness Becomes an Identity?" *The Cut*, July 24, 2019. www.thecut.com/2019 /07/what-happens-when-lyme-disease-becomes-an-identity.html.

- Fitts, Robert K. "The Archaeology of Middle-Class Domesticity and Gentility in Victorian Brooklyn." *Historical Archaeology* 33, no. 1 (1999): 39–62.

- Fleming, Amy. "Keep It Clean: The Surprising 130-year History of Handwashing." *The Guardian*, March 18, 2020. www.theguardian .com/world/2020/mar/18/keep-it-clean-the-surprising-130-year -history-of-handwashing.

- Ford, Brian J. *Single Lens: The Story of the Simple Microscope.* New York: HarperCollins, 1985.

- Fottrell, Quentin. "Coronavirus Has Killed More People Than SARS, But the Fatality Rate Is Still Far Lower—Here's Why That Could Change." *MarketWatch*, February 9, 2020. www.marketwatch.com /story/coronavirus-is-less-deadly-than-sars-but-that-may-explain -why-its-so-contagious-2020-01-30.

- Fournier, Alfred. *Syphilis and Marriage.* New York: D. Appleton, 1882.

- France, David. *How to Survive a Plague: The Story of How Activists and Scientists Tamed AIDS.* New York: Vintage, 2017.

- Fyfe, Aiyleen, and Bernard Lightman, eds. *Science in the Marketplace: Nineteenth-Century Sites and Experiences.* Chicago: University of Chicago Press, 2007.

- Gallagher, James. "Drug-Resistant Superbug Spreading in Europe's Hospitals." BBC News, July 29, 2019. www.bbc.com/news/health -49132425.

- Garrett, Elizabeth. *An Enquiry into the Character of the Contagious Disease Acts.* London: 1870.

- Garza, Lisa Maria. "Dallas Ebola Patient Vomited Outside Apartment on Way to Hospital." Reuters, October 1, 2014. https://jp .reuters.com/article/instant-article/idUSKCN0HP2F720141001.

- Gaulke, Mark, MD. Personal communication.

- "The Gay Divide." *The Economist* 413 (2014): 36.

- "The Germ Theory Again." *Chambers's Magazine*, November 1897.

- Gilbert, Kathy L. "Church Mourns Ebola Death of Sierra Leone Surgeon." *UMNews*, November 17, 2014. www.umnews.org/en/news /sierra-leone-surgeon-with-ebola-arrives-in-us.

- Gilbert, Pamela K. *Cholera and Nation: Doctoring the Social Body in Victorian England.* New York: SUNY Press, 2009.

- ———. *Mapping the Victorian Social Body.* New York: SUNY Press, 2004.

- ———. "On Cholera in Nineteenth-Century England." *BRANCH: Britain, Representation and Nineteenth-Century History*, edited by Dino Franco Felluga. Extension of Romanticism and Victorianism on the Net. www.branchcollective.org/?ps_articles=pamela-k-gilbert-on-cholera-in-nineteenth-century-england.

- Green, Edward C. *Rethinking AIDS Prevention: Learning from Successes in Developing Countries*. Westport: Praeger, 2003.

- Greenhow, Thomas Michael. *Cholera, as It Has Recently Appeared in Newcastle and Gateshead; Including Cases Illustrative of Its Physiology and Pathology, with a View to the Establishment of Sound Principles of Practice*. Philadelphia: Carey & Lea, 1832.

- Griffiths, Emma. "World's Untold Stories: Romania's Lost Children." CNN, November 23, 2007. https://www.cnn.com/CNNI/Programs/untoldstories/blog/2007/07/romania-little-boy-lost.html.

- Grundy, Isobel. *Lady Mary Wortley Montagu*. Oxford: Oxford University Press, 1999.

- "Guard Your Mouth Against Germs." Formamint advertisement, *The Tatler and Bystander* 59 (1913): 378.

- Hall, Stephanie. "Stories from the 1918–1919 Influenza Pandemic from Ethnographic Collections." Library of Congress, April 15, 2020. https://blogs.loc.gov/folklife/2020/04/stories-influenza-pandemic/.

- "Hall's Sanitary Washable Distemper, A New Sanitary Water Paint." Advertisement, *Strand Magazine* 18 (1899): xxxlx.

- Hallett, Christine. "The Attempt to Understand Puerperal Fever in the Eighteenth and Early Nineteenth Centuries: The Influence of Inflammation Theory." *Medical History* 49, no. 1 (2005): 1–28.

- Hamlin, Christopher. *Cholera: The Biography*. Oxford: Oxford University Press, 2009.

- Han, Xiang Y., and Francisco J. Silva. "On the Age of Leprosy." *PLOS Neglected Tropical Diseases* 8, no. 2 (2014).

- Harp, Jordan, PhD. Personal communication.

- *Harper's Weekly* 27, no. 1367 (1883): 42.

- Harris, Jonathan Gil. *Foreign Bodies and the Body Politic: Discourse of Social Pathology in Early Modern England*. Cambridge: Cambridge University Press, 1998.

- Hauge, Olav H. "Du Var Vinden." In Olav H. Hauge, *Vakraste Dikt*. Oslo: Samlaget, 2014.

- Healy, Margaret. "Defoe's Journal and the English Plague Writing Tradition." *Literature and Medicine* 22, no. 1 (2003): 25–44.

- Hempel, Sandra. "Obituary: John Snow." *The Lancet* 381, no. 9874 (2013).

- Hernandez, Dominic. "Fast Facts: Maternity Leave Policies Across the Globe." *Vital Record*, January 23, 2018. https://vitalrecord.tamhsc.edu/fast-facts-maternity-leave-policies-across-globe/.

- Higgins-Dunn, Noah, and Berkeley Lovelace Jr. "WHO Warns COVID Reinfections May Occur as Data Suggests Antibodies

Wane." CNBC, December 4, 2020. www.cnbc.com/2020/12/04/who-warns-covid-reinfections-may-occur-as-data-suggests-antibodies-wane.html.

- Hodge, Hugh L. *On the Non-contagious Character of Puerperal Fever.* Philadelphia: T. K. and P. G. Collins, 1852.

- Hogenboom, Melissa. "Ebola: Is Bushmeat Behind the Outbreak?" BBC News, October 19, 2014. www.bbc.com/news/health-29604204.

- Høie, Bent. Untitled talk and Facebook post, trans. Rachel Peterson, April 27, 2020. www.facebook.com/BentHoie/photos/a.16449877 3742538/1373854849473585/?type=3&theater.

- Hollar, Gladys, and Glenn Hollar. "Interview with Gladys and Glenn Hollar." Interview by Jacquelyn Hall, transcribed by Jean Houston. Carolina Piedmont Project, University of North Carolina at Chapel Hill Southern Oral History Program, 1980. https://exhibits.lib.unc.edu/files/original/b2ba2e31dcb2cad3823923299b3343ff.pdf.

- Holmes, Oliver Wendell. "The Contagiousness of Puerperal Fever." In *Medical Essays.* Cambridge: Riverside, 1891, 103–72.

- Hooker, Claire, Chris Degeling, and Paul Mason. "Dying a Natural Death: Ethics and Political Activism for Endemic Infectious Disease." In *Endemic: Essays in Contagion Theory.* Ed. Kari Nixon and Lorenzo Servitje. London: Palgrave, 2016, 265–90.

- Hurwitz, Brian, and Marguerite Dupree. "Why Celebrate Joseph Lister?" *Lancet* 379, no. 9820 (2012): 39–40, https://doi.org/10.1016/S0140-6736(12)60245-1.

- Hyslop, Leah. "Potted Histories: Kedgeree." *Telegraph*, July 10, 2013. www.telegraph.co.uk/foodanddrink/10157307/Potted-histories -kedgeree.html.

- Infectious Disease Society of America. "Ebola Facts." https://www .idsociety.org/public-health/ebola/ebola-resources/ebola-facts/.

- Ingram, Brooke. "The Many Presentations of Syphilis." *Dermatology Nurses' Association* 8, no. 5 (2016): 318–24.

- Institute of Urban Studies. "Vickery Meadow Strategic Plan." Issuu.com, August 9, 2018. https://issuu.com/institute-uta/docs/ vickery_meadow.

- "Izal Powder." *Strand Magazine*, January 1893.

- Jarussi, Loretta. "'He'll Come Home in a Box': the Spanish Influenza of 1918 Comes to Montana." Interview by Laurie Mercier, Montana Historical Society. History Matters: The U.S. Survey Course on the Web. http://historymatters.gmu.edu/d/14.

- Johansen, Frederick A. "Similarities in the Manifestations of Leprosy and Tuberculosis." *American Review of Tuberculosis* 35, no. 5, (1937): 609–17.

- Johnson, Garfield. "An Interview with Garfield Johnson." Interview by Ann Brantley, *Pandemic Influenza of 1918*, http://video1.adph .state.al.us/alphtn/pandemic/GarfieldJohnson/Local/transcript _garfieldjohnson.pdf.

- Johnson, Steven. "The Deadliness of the 2014 Ebola Outbreak Was Not Inevitable." *New York Times*, November 17, 2020. www

.nytimes.com/2020/11/17/books/review/fevers-feuds-and-diamonds
-paul-farmer.html.

- Johnson, Steven Ross. "CMS Finalizes Hospital Antibiotics Stewardship Requirements." *Modern Healthcare*, September 26, 2019. www.modernhealthcare.com/safety-quality/cms-finalizes-hospital -antibiotic-stewardship-requirements.

- Jordan, Douglas, Terrence Tumpey, and Barbara Jester. "The Deadliest Flu: The Complete Story of the Discovery and Reconstruction of the 1918 Pandemic Virus." Centers for Disease Control and Prevention, 2019. www.cdc.gov/flu/pandemic-resources/reconstruction-1918-virus .html.

- Juengel, Scott J. "Writing Decomposition: Defoe and the Corpse." *Journal of Narrative Technique* 25 (1995): 139–53.

- Kahan, Dan M. "Fixing the Communication Failure." *Nature* 463 (2010): 296–97. https://doi.org/10.1038/463296a.

- Kahan, Dan M., D. Braman, G. L. Cohen, J. Gastil, and P. Slovic. "Who Fears the HPV Vaccine, Who Doesn't, and Why? An Experimental Study of the Mechanisms of Cultural Cognition." *Law and Human Behavior* 34, no. 6 (2010): 501–16.

- Kahan, Dan M., Ellen Peters, Maggie Wittlin, Paul Slavic, Lisa L. Ouellette, Donald Braman, and Gregory Mandel. "The Polarizing Impact of Science Literacy and Numeracy on Perceived Climate Change Risks." *Scholarly Commons, Nature Climate Change* 2 (2012): 732–35. https://doi.org/10.1007/s10979-009-9201-0.

- Kahneman, Daniel, and Amos Tversky. "Prospect Theory: An Analysis of Decision Under Risk." *Econometrica* 47, no. 2 (1979): 263–92. https://doi.org/10.2307/1914185.

- Kapetanios Meir, Natalie. "'A Fashionable Dinner is Arranged as Follows': Victorian Dining Taxonomies." *Victorian Literature and Culture* 33, no. 1 (2005): 133–48.

- Kaplish, Lalita. "Happy Birthday John Snow." *Wellcome Collections* (blog), 2013.

- Karlamangla, Soumya. "Many Aren't Buying Public Officials' 'Stay-at-Home' Message. Experts Say There's a Better Way." *Los Angeles Times*, December 7, 2020. www.latimes.com/california/story/2020-12-07/coronavirus-stay-home-messaging-la-harm-reduction.

- Katic, Gordon, and Sam Fenn. "Secondary Symptoms #5: I Can't Breathe." *Cited* (podcast), June 6, 2020.

- Kazaura, Method R., and Rolv T. Lie. "Down's Syndrome and Paternal Age in Norway." *Paediatric and Perinatal Epidemiology* 16, no. 4, (2002): 314–19.

- Keating, Caitlin. "Ebola Survivor Amber Vinson: 'I Didn't Know If I Would Survive.'" *People*, November 6, 2014. https://people.com/celebrity/ebola-survivor-amber-vinson-i-didnt-know-if-i-would-survive/.

- Kelley, Alexandra. "COVID-19 Reinfections Likely as Antibody Counts Fall: WHO." *Hill*, December 4, 2020. https://thehill.com/changing-america/well-being/medical-advances/528828-covid-19-reinfections-likely-as-antibody-counts.

- "Kill Those Germs!" Vapex advertisement, *The Humorist* 21 (October 1932): 290.

- Kohn, George Childs., ed. *Encyclopedia of Plague and Pestilence: From Ancient Times to the Present.* 3rd ed. New York: Facts on File, 2008.

- Kristeva, Julia. *Powers of Horror: An Essay on Abjection.* New York: Columbia University Press, 1982.

- Kuhn, Thomas. *The Structure of Scientific Revolutions.* Chicago: University of Chicago Press, 1996.

- Latham, Baldwin. *The Utilisation of Sewage.* London: E and F. N., 1867.

- Lawlor, Christopher. *Consumption and Literature: The Making of a Romantic Disease.* Basingstoke, UK: Palgrave Macmillan, 2006.

- Layne, Tacy. "They Need to Cry." World Orphanages, April 20, 2016.

- Leavitt, Judith. *Brought to Bed: Childbearing in America 1750 to 1950.* New York: Oxford University Press, 1986.

- ———. *Typhoid Mary: Captive to the Public Health.* New York: Beacon, 1996.

- Leavy, Barbara Fass. *To Blight with Plague: Studies in a Literary Theme.* New York: New York University Press, 1992.

- Lee, Elmer. "Treatment of Asiatic Cholera." *JAMA* 1895, no. 25 (1895): 960–63. doi:10.1001/jama.1895.02430250008001b.

- Lerner, Barron H. "Searching for Semmelweis." *The Lancet* 383, no. 9913 (2014): 210–11. http:// doi.org/10.1016/s0140-6736(14) 60062-3.

- Levine, George. *Realism, Ethics and Secularism: Essays on Victorian Literature and Science.* New Brunswick, NJ: Rutgers University Press, 2009. https://doi.org/10.1017/CBO9780511484872.

- Liggins, Emma. "Writing against the 'Husband-Fiend': Syphilis and Male Sexual Vice in the New Woman Novel." *Women's Writing* 7 (2000): 175–95.

- Loewenstein, George F., Elke W. Weber, Christopher K. Hsee, and Ned Welch. "Risk as Feelings." *Psychological Bulletin* 127, no. 2 (2001): 267–86.

- Lopez-Martinez, Melissa. "Psychologist Hopes the Pandemic Can Help Reduce the Stigma Against OCD." CTV News, July 19, 2020. www.ctvnews.ca/health/psychologist-hopes-the-pandemic-can -help-reduce-the-stigma-against-ocd-1.5030557.

- Ludka-Gaulke, Tiffany, MD. Personal communication.

- Lytle, Alan. "Saving Stories: Firsthand Accounts of Spanish Flu Pandemic." WUKY, podcast audio, April 14, 2020. https://www .wuky.org/post/saving-stories-first-hand-accounts-spanish-flu -pandemic#stream/0.

- Ma, Y., C. R. Horsburgh Jr., L. F. White, and H. E. Jenkins. "Quantifying TB Transmission: A Systematic Review of Reproduction Number and Serial Interval Estimates for Tuberculosis." *Epidemiol Infect* 146, no. 12 (2018): 1478–94.

• Mackay, Ian M. "Ebola Virus in the Semen of Convalescent Men." *The Lancet: Infectious Diseases* 15, no. 2 (2015): 149–50.

• MacNeil, Adam, Philippe Glaziou, Charalambos Sismandis, Anand Date, Susan Maloney, and Katherine Floyd. "Global Epidemiology of Tuberculosis and Progress toward Meeting Global Targets Worldwide 2018." *Centers for Disease Control and Prevention: Morbidity and Mortality Weekly Report* 69, no. 11 (2020): 281–85.

• Malavaud, Sandra. "Hospital Cleaning, A Key Element to Prevent Cross-Transmission and Amplification of Antimicrobial-Resistant Disease Outbreak." AMR Control, July 12, 2016. http://resistancecontrol .info/2016/infection-prevention-and-control/hospital-cleaning-a-key -element-to-prevent-cross-transmission-and-amplification-of-anti microbial-resistant-disease-outbreaks/.

• Mandavilli, Apoorva. "Can You Get COVID-19 Again? It's Very Unlikely, Experts Say." *New York Times*, July 22, 2020. www.nytimes .com/2020/07/22/health/covid-antibodies-herd-immunity.html.

• Marcus, Julia. "Quarantine Fatigue Is Real." *Atlantic*, May 11, 2020. www.theatlantic.com/ideas/archive/2020/05/quarantine-fatigue -real-and-shaming-people-wont-help/611482/.

• Markel, Howard, Harvey B. Lipman, Alexander Navarro, Alexandra Sloan, Joseph R. Michalsen, Alexandra Minna Stern, and Martin S. Cetron. "Nonpharmaceutical Interventions Implemented by US Cities During the 1918–1919 Influenza Pandemic." *Journal of the American Medical Association* 298 (2007): 644–54.

- Marselas, Kimberly. "Flying Insects Likely to Spread Superbugs at Nursing Facilities." *McKnights*, June 25, 2019. www.mcknights.com /news/flying-insects-likely-to-spread-superbugs-at-nursing-facilities/.

- Marshall, Ashley. "Daniel Defoe as Satirist." *Huntington Library Quarterly* 70, no. 4 (2007): 553–76.

- Martin, Emily. *The Woman in the Body: A Cultural Analysis of Reproduction.* Boston: Beacon Press, 2001.

- Mathur, Rupal, MD. Personal communication.

- McDonald, Sarah. Personal communication.

- McDonnel, Gerald, and A. Denver Russell. "Antiseptics and Disinfectants: Activity, Action and Resistance." *Clinical Microbiology Reviews* (2001).

- Meier, Thomas Keith. *Defoe and the Defense of Commerce.* Victoria: University of Victoria Press, 1987.

- Metcalfe, Tom. "For the First Time, Scientists Detect the Ghostly Signal That Reveals the Engine of the Universe." NBC News, November 25, 2020.

- Mi, Sha, Xinhua Lee, Xiang-ping Li, Geertruida M. Veldman, Heather Finnerty, Lisa Racie, Edward LaVallie, Xiang-Yang Tang, Phillippe Edouard, Steve Howes, James C. Keith Jr., and John McCoy. "Syncytin Is a Captive Retroviral Envelope Protein Involved in Human Placental Morphogenesis." *Nature* 403 (2000): 785–89.

- Michaelis, Randy, PhD. Personal communication.

- Michaelson, Karen L. *Childbirth in America*. Connecticut: Praeger Publishing, 1988.

- Milkman, Katy. "Take the Deal!" *Choiceology* (podcast), season 4, episode 4, October 2019.

- Mody, Lona, et al. "Multidrug-Resistant Organisms in Hospitals: What Is On Patient Hands and in Their Rooms?" *Clinical Infectious Diseases* 69, no. 11 (2019): 1837–44. https://doi.org/10.1093/cid/ciz092.

- Mondelli, Mario U., Marta Colaneri, Elena M. Seminari, Fausto Baldanti, and Raffaele Bruno. "Low Risk of SARS-CoV-2 Transmission by Formites in Real-Life Conditions." *Lancet: Infectious Diseases* (2020). https://doi.org/10.1016/S1473-3099(20)30678-2.

- Montagu, Lady Mary Wortley. *The Turkish Embassy Letters*. Edited by Teresa Heffernan and Daniel O'Quinn. Ontario: Broadview, 2013.

- Mozes, Alan. "Study Finds Rise in Domestic Violence During COVID." WebMD, August 18, 2020. www.webmd.com/lung/news/20200818/radiology-study-suggests-horrifying-rise-in-domestic-violence-during-pandemic#1.

- Muzzi, Alba, Elena Seminari, Tiziana Feletti, Luigia Scudeller, Piero Marone, Carmine Tinelli, Lorenzo Minoli, Carlo Marena, Patrizia Mangiarotti, and Maurizio Strosseli. "Post-exposure Rate of Tuberculosis Infection Among Health Care Workers Measured with Tuberculin Skin Test Conversion after Unprotected Exposure to Patients with Pulmonary Tuberculosis: 6-Year Experience in an Italian Teaching Hospital." *BMC Infectious Diseases* 14 (2014): 324.

- Narain, Jai Prakash. "Responding to the Ebola Virus Disease in West Africa: Lessons for India." *Indian Journal of Medical Research* 141, no. 3 (2015): 263–65. https://pubmed.ncbi.nlm.nih.gov/25963484/.

- Narasimham, Padmanesan, James Wood, Chandini Raina MacIntyre, and Dilip Mathai. "Risk Factors for Tuberculosis." *Pulmonary Medicine* (2013).

- Nattrass, Nicoli. *The AIDS Conspiracy: Science Fights Back.* New York: Columbia University Press, 2012.

- Newman, Francis W. *The Cure of the Great Social Evil, with Special Reference to Recent Laws Delusively Called Contagious Diseases' Acts.* London: Trubner, 1869.

- Newsom, S. W. B. "The History of Infection Control: Cholera–John Snow and the Beginnings of Epidemiology." *Journal of Infection Prevention* 6, no. 6 (2005): 12–15.

- Newsom Kerr, M. L. *Contagion, Isolation, and Biopolitics in Victorian London.* London: Palgrave, 2018.

- "Memories of the 1918 Pandemic from Those Who Survived." *New York Times*, April 4, 2020. www.nytimes.com/2020/04/04/us/spanish -flu-oral-history.html.

- Niederhuber, Matthew. "The Fight over Inoculation during the 1721 Boston Smallpox Epidemic." *Harvard Science in the News: Special Edition on Infectious Disease*, December 31, 2014. http://sitn .hms.harvard.edu/flash/special-edition-on-infectious-disease/2014 /the-fight-over-inoculation-during-the-1721-boston-smallpox -epidemic/.

- Nixon, Kari, and Lorenzo Servitje. "An Ethics Debate for the Ages: American Individualism and the Dilemma of the Healthy Carrier." *American Literature* 92 (2020): 737–43.

- ———. *Endemic: Essays in Contagion Theory*. London: Palgrave, 2016.

- ———. "Grieving Our Collective Loss, One Stitch at a Time." *YES!*, May 1, 2020. www.yesmagazine.org/opinion/2020/05/01 /coronavirus-death-grief/.

- ———. "I'm a Mom and a Vaccine Researcher. Here's Why You Should Vaccinate Your Children." *HuffPost*, April 25, 2019. www .huffpost.com/entry/child-vaccinations-risk_n_5cb75091e4b0823 3dbddae6d.

- ———. "Keep Bleeding: Hemorrhagic Sores, Trade, and the Necessity of Leaky Boundaries in Defoe's *Journal of the Plague Year*." *Journal for Early Modern Cultural Studies* 14 (2014): 62–81.

- ———. *Kept from All Contagion: Germ Theory, Disease, and the Dilemma of Human Contact in Late Nineteenth-Century Literature*. Albany: SUNY University Press, 2020.

- ———. "Why I Wore Black after He Died." *YES!*, October 2, 2019. www.yesmagazine.org/issue/death/opinion/2019/10/02/grief-dying -mourning-victorian-culture/.

- Onishi, Norimitsu. "U.S. Patient Aided Pregnant Liberian, Then Took Ill." *New York Times*, October 1, 2014.

- "Oral Histories." Southern Oral History Program, UNC: Center for the Study of the American South, n.d. https://exhibits.lib.unc .edu/exhibits/show/going-viral/oral-histories.

- Otis, Laura. *Membranes: Metaphors of Invasion in Nineteenth-Century Literature, Science, and Politics.* Baltimore: Johns Hopkins University Press, 2000.

- Ott, Katherine. *Fevered Lives: Tuberculosis in American Culture since 1870.* Boston: Harvard University Press, 1999.

- "Passages from the Diary of a Late Physician: Consumption." Museum of Foreign Literature, January 1831.

- "The Patent Hygienic Ventilating Waterproof Coat." Advertisement, *Illustrated Sporting and Dramatic News* 6 (1877): 375.

- Paxson, Christina. "College Campuses Must Reopen in the Fall. Here's How We Do It." *New York Times*, April 26, 2020. www.nytimes.com/2020/04/26/opinion/coronavirus-colleges-universities.html.

- Pearson, Karl. *Tuberculosis, Heredity, and Environment.* London: Dulau and Co, Ltd., 1912.

- Peterson, Anne Helen. "Welcome the Covid Influencer." *Culture Study*, August 30, 2020. https://annehelen.substack.com/p/welcome-the-covid-influencer.

- Pfister, Eugene. "Plague Inc.—Designing Virtual Pandemics." Hypotheses.org, April 29, 2020. https://hccd.hypotheses.org/39.

- Pharis, James and Nannie. "Interview with James and Nannie Pharis." Interview by Allen Tullos, transcribed by David Knudsen. Piedmont Social History Project, University of North Carolina at Chapel Hill Southern Oral History Program, 1978. https:/

/exhibits.lib.unc.edu/files/original/803c69dfd9f63f7dd7ff699186e
7b93d.pdf.

- Phillips, Miles H. "The History of the Prevention of Puerperal Fever." *British Medical Journal* 1, no. 4017 (1938): 1–7.

- Poore, G. V. *Dry Methods of Sanitation.* London: Edward Stanford, 1894.

- Powell, Farran, and Emma Kerr. "What You Need to Know About College Tuition Costs." *U.S. News & World Report,* September 17, 2020. https://www.usnews.com/education/best-colleges/paying-for -college/articles/what-you-need-to-know-about-college-tuition-costs.

- Preston, Richard. *The Hot Zone: The Terrifying True Story of the Origins of the Ebola Virus.* New York: Anchor, 1993.

- "Pro and Con; or, Cholera or No Cholera?" *The Tatler* (1832): 173.

- Puntis, J. W. "Hugh Downman and Smallpox Inoculation." *Archives of Disease in Childhood* 88 (2003).

- Quetel, Claude. *History of Syphilis.* Translated by Judith Braddock and Brian Pike. Cambridge: Polity Press, 1990.

- "Recent Deaths." *Wesleyan-Methodist Magazine* (1832): 688.

- Register Boone, Edna. "An Interview with Edna Register Boone." *Pandemic Influenza of 1918,* n.d. http://video1.adph.state.al.us /alphtn/pandemic/EdnaBoone/Local/transcript_ednaboone.pdf.

- Reichler, Mary R., et al. "Risk and Timing of Tuberculosis among Close Contacts of Persons with Infectious Tuberculosis." *Journal of Infectious Disease* 218, no. 6 (2018): 1000–1008.

- Reynolds, Dr. Ernest V. "Interview." Interview by Mary Kasamatsu, Vermont History, Vermont Historical Society, March 24, 1988. https://vermonthistory.org/documents/GrnMtnChronTranscripts /200-20ReynoldsErnestV.pdf.

- Richetti, John. *Daniel Defoe*. Boston: Twayne Publishers, 1987.

- Robinson, Gurtys. "An Interview with Gurtys Robinson." Interview by Ann Brantley, *Pandemic Influenza of 1918*, http://video1.adph .state.al.us/alphtn/pandemic/gurtisrobinson/Local/transcript _gurtisrobinson.pdf.

- Rooks, Judith Pence. *Midwifery and Childbirth in America*. Philadelphia: Temple University Press, 1997.

- Roosen, William. *Daniel Defoe and Diplomacy*. Selinsgrove: Susquehanna University Press, 1986.

- Ross, Loretta, and Ricky Solinger. *Reproductive Justice: An Introduction*. Oakland: University of California Press, 2017.

- Rothman, Barbara Katz. *In Labor: Women and Power in the Birthplace*. New York: Norton, 1982.

- Rusnock, Andrea. "Historical Context and the Roots of Jenner's Discovery." *Human Vaccines and Immunotherapeutics* 12 (2016): 2025–28.

- ———. *Vital Accounts: Quantifying Health and Population in Eighteenth-Century England and France*. Cambridge: Cambridge University Press, 2009.

- Russell, William L. "Consumption: The Conditions Which Invite a Foothold of This Dread Disease." *Maine Farmer*, February 4, 1897.

- Rybicki, Ed. "Where Did Viruses Come From?" *Scientific American*, March 27, 2008. www.scientificamerican.com/article/experts-where -did-viruses-come-fr/.

- Sanchez, M. A., and S. M. Blower. "Uncertainty and Sensitivity Analysis of the Basic Reproductive Rate. Tuberculosis as an Example." *American Journal of Epidemiology* 145, no. 12 (1997): 1127–37.

- "Sanitas Destroys All Disease Germs." Advertisement, *The Sphere* 34 (1908).

- Sanlam Investments. "Prospect Theory (explained in a minute)." *Behavioral Finance*, May 13, 2016. YouTube video, 1:36. www.youtube .com/watch?v=sM91d5I36P.

- Sayles, A. "Caring for Little Ones Left Orphans by the Epidemic of Influenza." *Albany Evening Journal*, 1918. Influenza Encyclopedia. https://quod.lib.umich.edu/f/flu/07z0flu.0000.070/1/--caring-for -little-ones-left-orphans?page=root;rgn=full+text;size=125;view=im age;q1=orphan.

- Schmidt, Amy, PhD, PE. Personal communication.

- Schreiber, Werner. *Infection: Infectious Disease in the History of Medicine*. Basle: Hoffman-La Rouche, 1987.

- Seager, Nicholas. "Lies, Damned Lies, and Statistics: Epistemology and Fiction in Defoe's 'A Journal of the Plague Year.'" *Modern Language Review* 103, no. 3 (2008): 639–53.

- Sekine, Takuya, André Perez-Potti, Olga Rivera-Ballesteros, Kristoffer Strålin, Jean-Baptiste Gorin, Annika Olsson, Sian Llewellyn-Lacey, Habiba Kamal, Gordana Bogdanovic, Sandra Muschiol, David J.Wullimann, Tobias Kammann, Johanna Emgård, Tiphaine Parrot, and Elin Folkesson. "Robust T Cell Immunity in Convalescent Individuals with Asymptomatic or Mild COVID-19." *Cell* 183 (2020): 158–68.

- Semmelweis, Ignaz. *The Etiology, The Concept, and the Prophylaxis of Childbed Fever*. Translated by Frank Murphy, edited by Sherwin B. Nuland. Birmingham: Classics of Medicine Library, 1981.

- Servitje, Lorenzo. *Medicine Is War: The Martial Metaphor in Victorian Literature and Culture*. Albany: SUNY University Press, 2021.

- Shaw, George Bernard. Preface, *The Doctor's Dilemma*. New York: Penguin, 1957.

- Shaw, John. *Antiseptics in Obstetric Nursing*. London: H. K. Lewis, 1890.

- Shelomi, Martan. "Why Did Some Diseases Evolve to Kill Their Hosts?" *Forbes*, May 26, 2017. www.forbes.com/sites/quora/2017/05/26/why-did-some-diseases-evolve-to-kill-their-hosts/?sh=764703dd5323.

- Shepherd, Ninnie. "Interview with Ninnie Shepherd." Interview by Sadie W. Stidham, April 5, 1979. Louie B. Nunn Center for

Oral History, University of Kentucky Libraries, https://kentucky oralhistory.org/ark:/16417/xt7rr49g7c3b.

- Sherman, Michael. "The Flu Epidemic, 1918." Vermont History, Vermont Historical Society, https://vermonthistory.org/flu-epidemic -1918.

- Shorter, Edward. *A History of Women's Bodies*. New York: Basic Books, 1982.

- Shrewsbury, J. F. D. *A History of the Bubonic Plague in the British Isles*. Cambridge: Cambridge University Press, 1970.

- "Sierra Leone Loses Its 10th Doctor to Ebola Outbreak." CBS News, December 7, 2014.

- Sinclair, William J. *Semmelweis: His Life and Doctrine: A Chapter in the History of Medicine*. Manchester: Manchester University Press, 1909.

- Sloot, Rosa, Maarten F. Schim ven der Loeff, Peter M. Kouw, and Martien W. Borgdorff. "Risk of Tuberculosis after Recent Exposure. A 10-Year Follow-up Study of Contacts in Amsterdam." *American Journal of Respiratory and Critical Care Medicine* 190, no. 9 (2014).

- Slovic, Paul, and Daniel Västfjäll. "The More Who Die, the Less We Care: Psychic Numbing and Genocide." In *Imagining Human Rights*, edited by Susanne Kaul and David Kim, 55–68. Berlin: De Gruyter, 2015.

- Smith, Andrew. *Victorian Demons: Medicine, Masculinity, and the Gothic at the fin-de-siècle*. Manchester, UK: Manchester University Press, 2004.

- Smith, Issar. "Mycobacterium tuberculosis Pathogenesis and Molecular Determinants of Virulence." *Clinical Microbiology Reviews* 16, no. 3 (2003): 463–96.

- Smith, J. Anderson. "Immunity from Disease." *Wesleyan-Methodist Magazine*, June 1893.

- Snow, John. *On the Mode of Communication of Cholera.* London: John Churchill, 1855.

- Sontag, Susan. *Illness as Metaphor.* New York: Farrar, Straus, and Giroux, 1978.

- "Southall's Sanitary Towels." Advertisement, *Strand Magazine* 18 (1899): vii.

- Sparham, Legard. *Reasons against the Practice of Inoculating the Small-Pox.* London: Peele, 1722.

- Spencer, Thomas. *On the Quality of the New River Company's Water.* London: Gilbert and Rivington, 1855.

- Spongberg, Mary. *Feminizing Venereal Disease: The Body of the Prostitute in Nineteenth-Century Medical Discourse.* New York: New York University Press, 1997.

- Stewardson, Andrew, and Didier Pittet. "Ignac Semmelweis—Celebrating a Flawed Pioneer of Patient Safety." *The Lancet* 378, no. 9785 (2011): 22–23. https://doi.org/10.1016/s0140-6736(11)61007-6.

- Stroman, Elissa. "South Plains Voices of the 1918 Influenza Pandemic." *Lubbock Avalanche-Journal*, April 25, 2020. www.lubbock

online.com/lifestyle/20200425/south-plains-voices-of-1918-influenza
-pandemic.

- Sudan, Rajani. *The Alchemy of Empire: Abject Materials and the Technologies of Colonialism*. New York: Fordham University Press, 2016.

- ———. *Fair Exotics: Xenophobic Subjects in English Literature, 1720–1850*. Philadelphia: University of Pennsylvania Press, 2002.

- "Syphilitic Child." Wellcome Images. Taken from Franz Mracek, *Atlas of Syphilis and the Venereal Diseases*. London: Rebman, 1898.

- Szabo, Liz, and Hannah Recht. "The Other COVID Risks: How Race, Income, ZIP Code Influence Who Lives or Dies." KHN, April 22, 2020. https://khn.org/news/covid-south-other-risk-factors-how
-race-income-zip-code-influence-who-lives-or-dies/.

- Szreter, Simon. *Health and Wealth: Studies in History and Policy*. Rochester, NY: University of Rochester Press, 2007.

- Taasaas, Rachel. Personal communication.

- Tansey, E. M. "From Germ Theory to 1945." In *Western Medicine: An Illustrated History*, edited by Irvine Loudon, 102–22. Oxford: Oxford University Press, 1997.

- Taub, Amanda. "A New Covid-19 Crisis: Domestic Abuse Rises Worldwide." *New York Times*, April 6, 2020. www.nytimes.com
/2020/04/06/world/coronavirus-domestic-violence.html.

- Taylor, Beck A. "Inaugural Address." Whitworth University, October 10, 2010. www.whitworth.edu/cms/administration/president-beck-a -taylor/speeches-and-messages/inaugural-address/.

- Taylor, Charles Bell. *Observations on the Contagious Disease Acts.* Nottingham, 1869.

- Taylor, Lisa. "Pandemic: A Woman on Duty." Library of Congress, March 26, 2020. https://blogs.loc.gov/folklife/2020/03/pandemic -a-woman-on-duty/?loclr=blogflt.

- "TB Is a Pandemic." TB Alliance, n.d. https://www.tballiance.org /why-new-tb-drugs/global-pandemic#:~:text=TB%20is%20 a%20Pandemic&text=Tuberculosis%20(TB)%20is%20a%20 global,infected%20with%20Mycobacterium%20tuberculosis%20(M.

- Tennyson, Alfred Lord. "The Lady of Shalott." 1832.

- Tharoor, Ishan. "The Pandemic Strengthens the Case for Universal Basic Income." *Washington Post,* April 9, 2020. www.washingtonpost .com/world/2020/04/09/pandemic-strengthens-case-universal -basic-income/.

- Thompson, Derek. "Hygiene Theater Is a Huge Waste of Time." *Atlantic,* July 27, 2020. www.theatlantic.com/ideas/archive/2020/07 /scourge-hygiene-theater/614599/.

- Thompson, James A. "Disentangling the Roles of Maternal and Paternal Age on Birth Prevalence of Down Syndrome and Other Chromosomal Disorders Using a Bayesian Modeling Approach." *BMC Medical Research Methodology* 19, no. 1 (2019): 82, doi: 10.1186/s12874-019-0720-1.

- Timberg, Craig, and Daniel Halperin. *Tinderbox: How the West Sparked the AIDS Epidemic and How the World Can Finally Overcome It.* London: Penguin Press, 2012.

- Tomes, Nany. *The Gospel of Germs: Men, Women, and the Microbe in American Life.* Cambridge: Harvard University Press, 1999.

- Tomes, N. J., and J. H. Warner. *Rethinking the Reception of the Germ Theory of Disease.* Special issue, *Journal of the History of Medicine* 52 (1997).

- Townsley, Jeramy, Karen Comer, and Matt Nowlin. "Socioeconomic Factors Explain Why Some New York ZIP Codes Were Hit Hardest by COVID-19." SAVI, June 24, 2020. www.savi.org/2020/06/24 /socioeconomic-factors-explain-why-some-new-york-zip-codes -were-hit-hardest-by-covid-19/.

- Troh, Louise. *My Spirit Took You In: The Romance That Sparked an Epidemic of Fear: A Memoir of the Life and Death of Thomas Eric Duncan, America's First Ebola Victim.* New York: Weinstein Publishing, 2015.

- ———. "The Tragic Love Story Behind America's First Ebola Victim." *Vanity Fair*, April 23, 2015. www.vanityfair.com/culture /2015/04/my-spirit-took-you-in-louise-troh-excerpt.

- Trotter, David. *Circulation: Defoe, Dickens and the Economics of the Novel.* New York: St. Martin's Press, 1988.

- Tseng, Chic-Peng, and Yu-Jiun Chan. "Overview of Ebola Virus Disease in 2014." *Journal of the Chinese Medical Association* 78, no. 1 (2015): 51–55.

- Tumlinson, Caitlin, MS NBCT. Personal communication.

- UNICEF. "Early Childhood Development and COVID-19." Unicef .org, April 2020. https://data.unicef.org/topic/early-childhood -development/covid-19/.

- VanArsdel, Rosemary, and J. Don Vann, ed. *Victorian Periodicals and Victorian Society*. Toronto: University of Toronto Press, 1995.

- Vapo-Cresolene Vaporizer, product box.

- "Vegetable Villains." *Good Words*, December 1883.

- Vinson, Jenna, and Clare Daniel. "'Power to Decide' Who Should Get Pregnant: A Feminist Rhetorical Analysis of Neoliberal Visions of Reproductive Justice." *Present Tense* 8, (2020). www .presenttensejournal.org/volume-8/power-to-decide-who-should -get-pregnant-a-feminist-rhetorical-analysis-of-neoliberal-visions -of-reproductive-justice/.

- Voss, Barbara L. "The Archaeology of Serious Games: Play and Pragmatism in Victorian-Era Dining." *American Antiquity* 84, no. 1 (2018): 26–47. https://doi.org/10.1017/aaq.2018.72.

- W. C. "The Germ Theory." *Chambers's Journal of Popular Literature, Science, and Art*, March 4, 1876.

- Wagstaffe, W. *A Letter to Dr. Friend Shewing the Danger and Uncertainty of Inoculating the Small Pox*. London: Butler, 1722.

- Wald, Priscilla. *Contagious: Cultures, Carriers, and the Outbreak Narrative*. Durham, NC: Duke University Press, 2008.

- Walkowitz, Judith. *Prostitution and Victorian Society: Women, Class, and the State.* Cambridge: Cambridge University Press, 1980.

- Wall, Cynthia. "Novel Streets: The Rebuilding of London and Defoe's 'A Journal of the Plague Years.'" *Studies in the Novel* 30, no. 2 (1998): 164–77.

- Weir, Kirsten. "The Lasting Impact of Neglect." *American Psychological Association* 45, no. 6, (2014): 36.

- Wertheim, Heiman F. L., Peter Horby, and John P. Woodall. *Atlas of Human Infectious Diseases.* Hoboken, NJ: Blackwell Publishing, 2012.

- Wertz, Richard W., and Dorothy C. Wertz. *Lying-In: A History of Childbirth in America.* New Haven, CT: Yale University Press, 1989.

- Wessner, David R. "How Did Viruses Evolve? Are They a Streamlined Form of Something That Existed Long Ago, or an Ultimate Culmination of Smaller Genetic Elements Joined Together?" *Scitable by Nature Education,* 2010. www.nature.com/scitable/topicpage/the-origins-of-viruses-14398218/.

- "West Nile Virus." New York State Department of Health, September 2017. www.health.ny.gov/diseases/west_nile_virus/fact_sheet.htm.

- Whitehead, Henry. "The Broad Street Pump: An Episode in the Cholera Epidemic of 1854." *Macmillan's Magazine* (1865): 113.

- Windsor, Matt. "Your ZIP Code Is a Risk Factor for COVID-19: Study Will Identify Where Testing, Therapies Are Needed Most."

UAB Reporter, October 19, 2020. www.uab.edu/reporter/research /discoveries-innovations/item/9297-your-zip-code-is-a-risk-factor-for -covid-19-study-will-identify-where-testing-therapies-are-needed-most.

- Woodville, William. *Reports of a Series of Inoculations for the Variola Vaccine or Cow-pox.* London: James Phillips and Son, 1799.

- World Health Organization. "Ebola Virus Disease—Democratic Republic of the Congo." WHO, July 25, 2018. www.who.int/csr /don/25-july-2018-ebola-drc/en/.

- ———. "What We Know About Transmission of the Ebola Virus among Humans." WHO, October 6, 2014. www.who.int/news /item/06-10-2014-what-we-know-about-transmission-of-the -ebola-virus-among-humans.

- Yong, Ed. "Some Microbes Have Been with Us Since Before We Existed." *Atlantic*, July 22, 2016. www.theatlantic.com/science/ar chive/2016/07/some-microbes-have-been-with-us-since-before-we -existed/492503/.

- Young, Michael E. "Hope Blooms in Vickery Meadow." *Dallas Morning News*, January 7, 2006. https://web.archive.org/web /20071208195906/http://www.dallasnews.com/sharedcontent /dws/news/localnews/stories/010806dnmetvickery.2a4bd98.html.

- Zelt, Mara, MS. Personal communication.

- "Zoetrope Strips: Milton Bradley." Stephen Herbert, n.d. www .stephenherbert.co.uk/zoetropestripsBradley.htm.

INDEX

INDEX

INDEX

INDEX

disease(s). *See also* sexually transmitted
diseases (STDs); individual names of
diseases
accounts of losing a loved one from,
14–15
affecting humans, xvi–xvii
author's interest in, xv–xvi
as caused by filth, 59–60
cultural biases on origins of, 10–11
filth correlated with, 60–61
as a given, xv
identifiable, 89–90, 177–78
making decisions on combatting, 85–87
naming. *See* naming practices
noxious airs believed to be cause of, 92
prejudice allowing spread of, 207–8
shaping how we conceptualize our
identities and communities, 88
social biases and spread of, 187–93
society's confusion about, 179–81
spread of. *See* spread of disease
study of past, in medical humanities,
xxiii–xiv
subtle and slow, 177–78, 179–80
transmission of. *See* transmission of
diseases
visible markings of a, 89–90, 177–78
visually noticeable, 177–78
Western medicine's war against,
xvii–xviii
disease language, spread of disease and,
187–93
disease management. *See* germ management;
risk elimination; sanitation theater
DNA, viruses and human, xx–xxi
doctors
accounts of losing loved ones from
disease by, 14–15
debate over puerperal fever, 79–80
Dublin, 1721, 3–5
maternal deaths and, 72, 73, 74
opposition to ideas and recommendations
about handwashing, 81–82
domestic violence, 165–66
Doughty, Caitlin, 108

"Dover Beach" (Arnold), 147, 148
Dowling, Linda, 188
Dublin, Ireland (1842), 2–5
Dubos, Jean, 179–80
Dubos, Rene, 179–80
Due Preparations for the Plague (Defoe), 19,
20, 22–23, 30, 51, 51n25
Duffield, Alice L. Mikel, 154n4
Duncan, Dr. James, 4–5
Duncan, Thomas Eric, 197–98
Durbach, Nadja, 12

E

East India Company, 9
Ebola virus
as endemic versus epidemic, 200
case of Thomas Eric Duncan, 197–98
fear reaction and, 205–7
in *The Hot Zone* (Preston), 194–95,
203–5
lessons learned from 2014 "outbreak,"
195
mortality rate, 196–97
as safe from the Western world, 201
studying origins of, 11
transmission of, 185, 196
as visible, 135
xenophobia and, 205–7
economic stimulus, 31
economy(ies)
Defoe's ideas about "flow" in, 33–34, 35
need for a free market, 33–34
public health ethics and, 139
risk elimination during plagues and, 46
education
examining role of free public, 166–68
higher, 169–71
school shut-downs and reopenings, 162,
164, 166, 167
elective surgeries, 121
emetics, 3
emotional reactions
risk assessment and, 49–50
risk elimination and, 52–53
endemic disease(s), 200–202

INDEX

England. *See also* London, England; Victorian era
  appearance of cholera in, 58–59
  idea of inoculations in (1721), 8–9
  Sunderland cholera outbreak (1832) in, 62–64
engrafting. *See* inoculation
Enlightenment, the, 44, 127
environmentalism, 66
epidemics. *See also* names of specific epidemics
  attitude toward, in the West, 201
  bias in locating sources of, 10–11
  Ebola virus as an, 200
  lack of preparation for, xxii
  nonpharmaceutical interventions used during, 29
  reassessing human interactions from, xxi
epidemiological spread. *See* spread of disease
epidemiology
  finding a "source" of contagion, 202–3
  John Snow as father of, 60
  as a "normalizing" science, 189
  social bias in research design, 10–11
Epstein, Steven, 189
essential workers, 16, 37
ethics. *See also* public health and public health ethics
  healthy carriers and, 133–34, 136–38
  personal liberties versus public's rights and, 134, 135–37
  personal versus shared realities and, 139–41

F

facts
  communicating through narrative versus, 82–83
  cultural biases versus, 184–85
  fluidity of, 129–30
  group acceptance chosen over, 84
"fake news," 144
Farr, William, 67
fear(s). *See also* denial-panic cycle; xenophobia

COVID-19 and, 206
  of death, 100, 107, 207
  risk assessment and, 49
  of social and emotional losses, 52–53
fecal matter, transmission of GI bugs through, 58
fecal transplants, 103
filth, connection between disease and, 59–61
Fischer, Molly, 131
"flattening the curve," 47, 163–64
fluidity
  of data, 42–43, 82
  in the economy, 33–34, 35
  of facts, 129–30
food delivery, contactless, 18, 29–30
Fort Smith, Arkansas (1915), 153–54
free market capitalism, 33–34
funeral industry, 108–9
funeral procession, during 1918 influenza pandemic, 155–56

G

garden mentality, 103, 104, 127
Gatlin, Agnes, 163
germ management. *See also* risk elimination; sanitation theater
  cure-all products during Victorian era, 122–25
  current day products for, 125
  finding the middle zone for, 103–4
  germ theory's influence on, 93–94
  OCD and, 97–98
  products advertised for, 96
  use of good bacteria for, 103
  whack-a-mole fallacy and, 97, 99–100
germ theory
  changing beliefs about risk elimination, 97
  contagion concept and, 89–90, 177
  development of, 89–90
  effect on understandings of identity and community, 90
  Ignaz Semmelweis and, 73–74
  influence on germ management, 93
  influencing attitudes about death, 95–96
  issues of power and authority and, 93–94

INDEX

North Carolina, 1918 influenza pandemic in, 157, 159–60
Norway, 35
novel, first English language, 19
novel coronavirus. *See also* COVID-19 pandemic
    antibiotic resistance and, 102
    healthy carriers, 135
    incubation period, 135, 197
    learning from others by studying historical figures of, xxv
    sanitation theater and, 101–2
    slow incubation time, 197
    use of term, xix
null hypotheses, 91

O

obsessive-compulsive disorder, 97–98
One Health, 65–66, 89, 101
open flow metaphor, 33
orphans and orphanages, 149–50
Otis, Laura, 93, 142, 143

P

panaceas, 122–27
pandemics. *See* Covid-19 pandemic; novel coronavirus
panic, cycle of denial and, 41–42, 44, 49–50, 113, 205–6
Pasteur, Louis, 73, 90
paternal age, Down syndrome pregnancy and, 130
pathogens. *See also* bacteria; disease(s); viruses
    bloodborne, 186, 191–92
    characteristics of a "subtle," 177
    existing without people, xvi–xvii
    prejudice and spread of, 207–8
    of tuberculosis, 178
Pearson, Karl, 180, 180*n*6
penicillin, 182
Pennsylvania, 1918 influenza pandemic in, 158–59
petri dish, 91
Petri, Julius, 91
phage therapy, 36

Pharis, James, 152, 158*n*10, 159*n*14
Pharis, Nannie, 158*n*10, 159*n*14
phase-of-life characteristics, 150–51
Philadelphia, Pennsylvania, 158–59
plague(s)
    Daniel Defoe writing about, 18, 19–26, 28–33, 38–39, 41, 42, 43–47, 51
    diseases from the past helping to prepare for future, xx, xxii, xxiv–xxv
    learning stories of people who lived through, xxiv–xxv
    1347 bubonic, xviii
Plague Inc., 177
polarization, 27, 75–76, 84, 144, 212
polio, 201
political extremes, 42
poor, the
    Defoe on handling, 30
    tuberculosis deaths and, 192
    vaccination debate and, 12–13
Portsmouth, UK (1873), 173–74
poverty. *See* class differences; poor, the
prejudice(s)
    allowing spread of disease, 187–88, 189–90, 207–8
    HIV and, 188–89, 191
    sexually transmitted diseases and, 181–83
    in statistics, 10–11
Presbyterian Hospital, Dallas, Texas, 197, 198
Preston, Richard, 194*n*1, 195, 196, 200, 203–7
probiotics, xx
prospect theory, 85–87
"psychic numbing," 40, 41
psychology
    antibiotic life and, 52
    "psychic numbing," 40
    psychological preparedness for COVID-19, 161–62
    rational emotive behavior therapy (REBT), 113–14
    risk elimination and, 52–53, 97–98
psychometrics, 38
public health and public health ethics

INDEX

crisis-care ethics, 14, 135, 138
Defoe on private interests and, 46
healthy carriers narrative and, 133–34,
136–38, 140
individual needs versus collective goals,
13–14, 26, 135–36
mandatory quarantines and, 26, 27
personal versus shared realities and,
139–41
recommendations, as polarizing, 84
public schooling, examining role of, 166–68
public service announcements (PSAs), 88
puerperal fever, 72–73, 79–80, 179

Q

quantitative research, 10–11, 178
quarantines
colleges/universities and, 169–71
Defoe on ineffectiveness of mandatory,
22–26, 29
delay in, 27, 29–30
domestic violence and, 165–66
enforcement of American mandatory, 28
impact on children during COVID-19,
164–65
individual versus public's needs and, 135
resistance to forced, during COVID
pandemic, 26–27
school closings and reopenings, 162, 164,
166, 167–69
of Typhoid Mary, 137–38, 146

R

racial biases and prejudices, 137, 197–98
racial protests (2020), 80–81
Radiology (journal), 165
realities, differing, 144
REBT (rational emotive behavior therapy),
113–14
religion
memento mori and, 106
secularization and, 98
turning to science instead of, 127–28
remote learning, 164–65, 166, 167, 168
research

John Snow's cholera, 60–61
quantitative, 10–11, 178
by Semmelweis, 72, 74
Reynolds, Ernest V., 155–56
risk(s)
human contact associated with, 64
middle ground for, 52
prospect theory and, 85–87
statistics and, 49–50
taking middle ground with, 51–52, 104
viewed from a perspective of losses versus
gains, 87
risk assessment, 48–50
risk aversion, 100, 102, 127, 162, 205
risk elimination. *See also* sanitation theater
"antibiotic life," 51, 52
antibiotic resistance and, 101–3
germ theory changing beliefs about, 97
as not possible, 38–41, 47, 97–98
problems with, 46, 52–53
statistics and, 49, 50
vigilance fatigue, 50
whack-a-mole fallacy and, 97, 99–100
risk mitigation, 47–48, 51–52, 100, 216.
See also masks and mask-wearing;
nonpharmaceutical interventions;
quarantines; social distancing
rituals, death, 100, 108, 109–10
Robinson Crusoe (Defoe), 19
Robinson, Gurtys, 163

S

sanitation movement, Victorian, 92–93
sanitation theater, 52. *See also* germ
management; handwashing; risk
elimination
antibiotic resistance, 102–3
denial of death and, 100, 109
during Ebola outbreak, Dallas, Texas,
199–200
fantasy of germ whack-a-mole, 98–99
novel coronavirus and, 102
path of moderation for, 103–4
Vienna, Austria (1847), 68–72
SARS (severe acute respiratory syndrome), 11

INDEX

ABOUT THE AUTHOR

Kari Nixon is a professor specializing in social reactions to infectious diseases. She works at Whitworth University, where she teaches about social responses to contagion and quarantine in medical humanities and Victorian literature courses. Her work on public health has been published for lay audiences in *HuffPost* and *YES!* magazine and on CNN.com. Her academic book, *Kept from All Contagion: Germ Theory, Disease, and the Dilemma of Human Contact*, published by SUNY University Press, tracks the social history of humankind's responses to disease in Victorian literature and popular culture. She regularly teaches about zombies, medical ethics, the problematic pressures on the health care system, and social justice issues for marginalized races and genders. She has edited numerous books on diseases in society. She lives in Washington State with her family.

INDEX

universal basic income, 31
universities and colleges, 169–71

V

vaccines and vaccinations, xviii. *See also*
 inoculation
 debate over individual rights versus
  collective good and, 13–14, 134
 mothers' hesitancy on, 15–16
 polio, 201
 resistance to compulsory, 12–13
 secondary infections from, 12, 16
 smallpox, 9, 12
 waiting for development of, 160–61
Veda Lux boutique, Spokane, WA, 111
venereal diseases. *See* sexually transmitted
 diseases (STDs)
Vermont, 1918 influenza pandemic in, 155–56
Vickery Meadow, Dallas, Texas, 198–99
Victorian era
 anesthesia used during, 121–22
 binary view of sexuality in, 188
 carbolic acid used during, 121–22,
  122n1, 123
 on cause of disease as filth, 59–60
 cholera's impact on, 59
 Contagious Disease Acts, 181–83
 death rituals, 109–10
 funeral industry, 108
 laws on sex workers, 181–83, 185
 medical cure-all products during, 122–25
 medical panaceas, 122–25
 objection to handwashing, 78–79
 overvalorization of science in, 127–28
 puerperal fever, debate on, 79–80, 80n9
 sanitary movement, 52, 92–93
 syphilis during, 181–82, 187–88
 tuberculosis during, 175–77, 178, 192
Vienna General Hospital, 68–72
Vinson, Amber, 199
Vinson, Jenna, 17
viruses. *See also* disease(s); Ebola virus; novel
 coronavirus
 computer, 143
 HIV, 183, 185, 186, 188, 189, 191–93

humans developed in tandem with, xx–xxi
norovirus, 58
treatment, 198
visible markings of a disease, 89–90, 177–78

W

Wald, Priscilla, 62, 136n4, 137, 202
Walkowitz, Judith, 174n1
waterborne source of cholera, 60, 61
wealth(y). *See also* class differences
 disease survival, 5
 Ebola "outbreak," Dallas, Texas, and,
  199–200
 vaccination scars and, 12
Western science, locating epidemic origins in
 non-Western spaces, 10–11. *See also*
 germ theory
West Nile virus, 202
"whack-a-mole" fallacy, 97–98, 99–100,
 102, 125
Whitehead, Henry, 53, 54, 54n1, 56–58, 61
Whitworth University, 51, 104, 169
Williams, Annie Laurie, 163
women. *See also* mothers and motherhood
 in accounts of losing a loved one, 14–15
 Contagious Disease Acts, 181–83
 lesson on listening to, 10–11
 in Lock Hospitals for having syphilis,
  173–74, 182
 nurse during 1918 influenza pandemic,
  153–55
 puerperal fever, 79–80
 sex workers, 181–83, 185, 201
 smallpox inoculation and, 1–2, 5–10,
  11–12
 Victorians on fear and worry in, 74
Woodhall, Louisa, 63–64
World War I, 154–55
World Wide Web, 142–43
Wuhan, China, xviii

X

xenophobia
 in Defoe's work, 46
 Ebola virus and, 200–201, 205–7